TO DIET

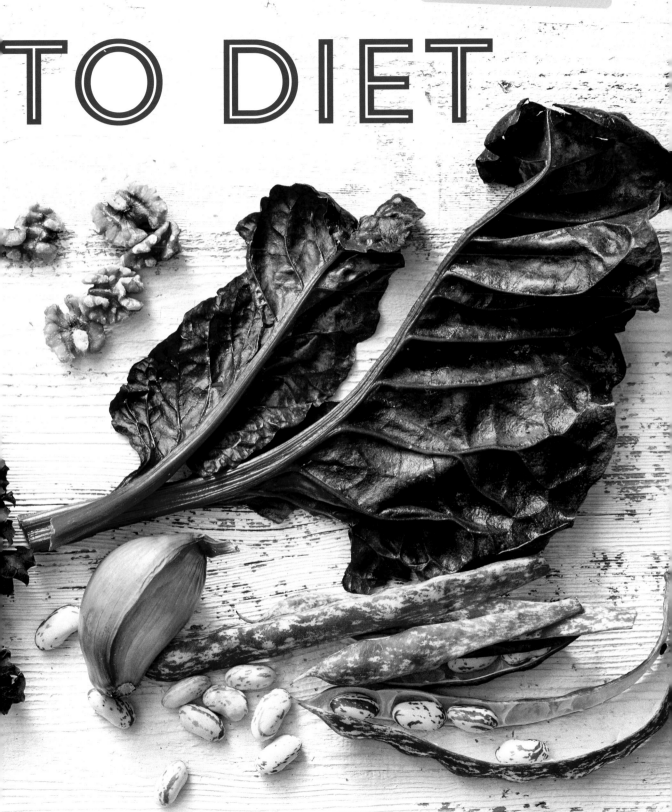

First published 2020 by Flatiron Books, New York

This paperback edition first published in the UK in 2021 by Bluebird,
an imprint of Pan Macmillan
The Smithson, 6 Briset Street, London EC1M 5NR

EU representative: Macmillan Publishers Ireland Ltd, 1st Floor,
The Liffey Trust Centre, 117–126 Sheriff Street Upper,
Dublin 1, D01 YC43

Associated companies throughout the world
www.panmacmillan.com

ISBN 978-1-5290-5924-3

1 3 5 7 9 8 6 4 2

A CIP catalogue record for this book is available from
the British Library.

Produced by Print Matters Productions, Inc.
Photography by Antonis Achilleos
Cover design by Jason Gabbert
Interior design by Alison Lew / Vertigo Design NYC

Printed and bound in China.

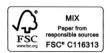

Visit **www.panmacmillan.com** to read more about all our books and to buy them. You will
also find features, author interviews and news of any author events, and you can sign up for
e-newsletters so that you're always first to hear about our new releases.

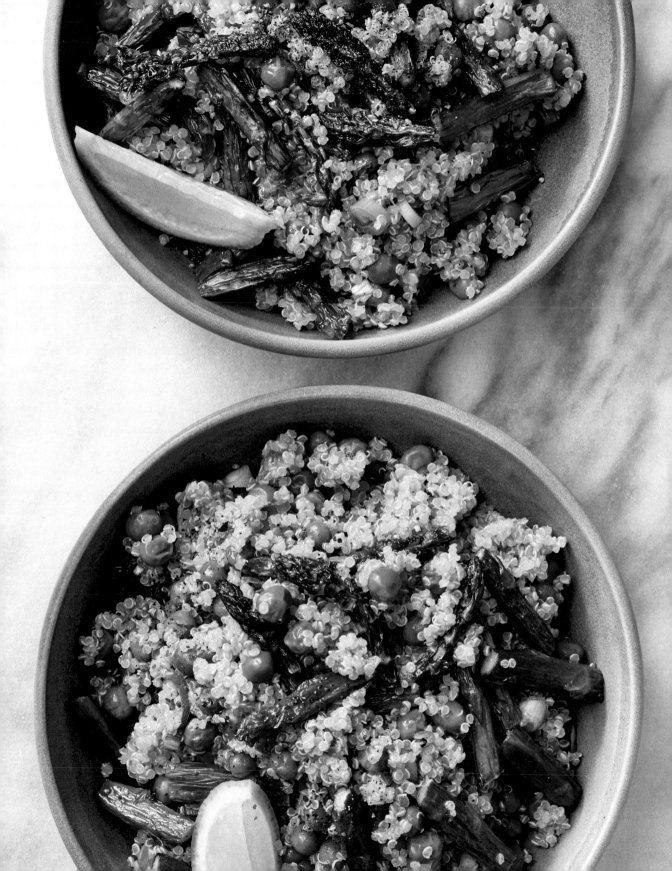

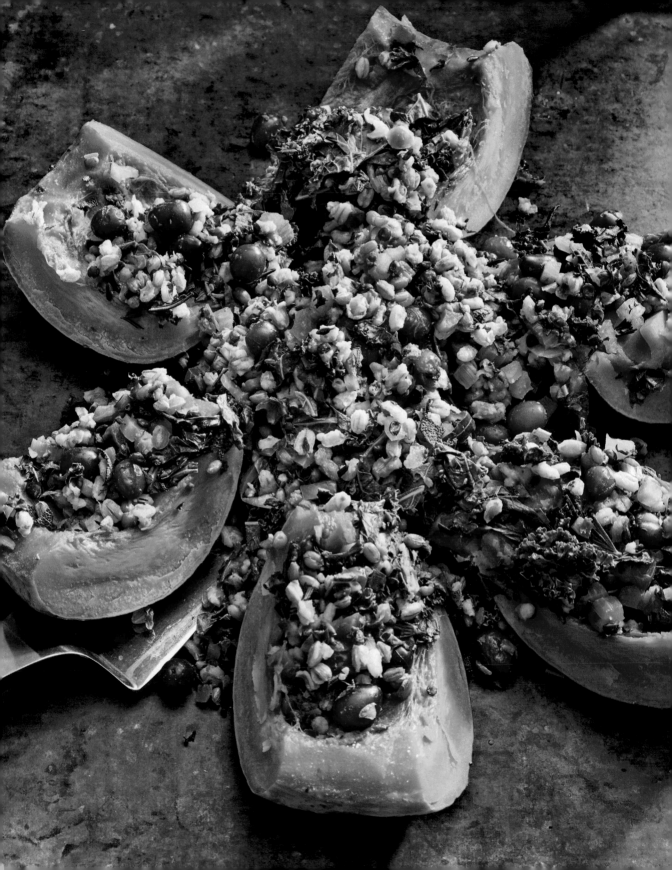

CONTENTS

INTRODUCTION

Surely, if there was a safe, simple, side-effect-free solution to the obesity epidemic, we would know about it by now, right? I'm not so sure. It may take an average of seventeen years before research evidence makes it into day-to-day clinical practice.[1]

Take one example that was particularly poignant for my family: heart disease. Decades ago, Dr Dean Ornish and his colleagues published evidence in one of the most prestigious medical journals in the world that our leading cause of death could be reversed with diet and lifestyle changes alone[2] – yet hardly anything changed.[3] Even now, hundreds of thousands of Americans continue to needlessly die each year from what we learned decades ago was a reversible condition.

I had seen it with my own eyes. My grandmother was cured of her end-stage heart disease by one of Dr Ornish's contemporaries, Nathan Pritikin, using similar methods. She had been given her medical death sentence at age sixty-five after one too many open-heart surgeries, but thanks to a healthy diet was able to live another thirty-one years – until she was ninety-six – to enjoy her six grandkids, including me.

So, if effectively the cure to our number one killer of men and women could get lost down a rabbit hole and ignored, what else might there be buried in the medical literature that could help my patients but just didn't have a corporate budget driving its promotion?

I made it my life's mission to find out.

That's why I became a doctor in the first place and why I started my nonprofit site, NutritionFacts.org. Everything on the website is free. There are no ads, no corporate sponsorships. It's strictly noncommercial; nothing is for sale.

I launched it as a public service, as a labour of love, as a tribute to my grandmother. New videos and articles are uploaded almost every day on the latest in evidence-based nutrition.

So, what does the science show is the best way to *lose weight*?

THE HOW NOT TO DIET APPROACH

I'm so sick and tired of the nutritional nonsense that comes out of the diet industry, feeding us an endless parade of quick-fix fads that always sell because they always fail. Repeat customers are their whole business model, yet people just line right back up to be fooled again.

The weight-loss industry is so corrupted by financial and ideological conflicts of interest that you can never know who to trust. Too often in diet books, the rule is to obfuscate rather than illuminate, cherry-picking facts to push some pet theory and ignoring the rest to promote their own agenda. It's the opposite of science. In true scholarship, your conclusions follow from the evidence, not the other way around.

I'm not interested in offering duelling anecdotes, and the last thing we need is more dietary dogma. What I am interested in is the science. When it comes to making life-and-death decisions as important as what to feed yourself and your family, as far as I'm concerned, there's only one question: *What does the best available balance of evidence say right now?*

My goal was to create the oxymoron: an evidence-based diet book.

The problem is that even just sticking to peer-reviewed medical literature is not enough as, concluded a commentary in the *New England Journal of Medicine*, 'False and scientifically unsupported beliefs about obesity are pervasive'[4] – even in scientific journals. The only way to get at the truth, then, is to dive deep into the primary literature and read all the original studies. Who's got time for that, though? There are more than half a million scientific papers on the subject with a hundred new ones published every day. Even researchers in the field might not be able to keep track of what's going on beyond their narrow domain. But that's what we do at NutritionFacts.org. We comb through tens of thousands of studies a year, so you and your doctors don't have to.

A DIET BOOK ABOUT NOT DIETING

Diets don't work by definition. Going on a diet implies that, at some point, you will go off the diet. Short-term fixes are no match for long-term problems. Lifelong weight control requires lifelong lifestyle changes.

First, a diet has to be sustainable. Consider water-only fasting. No diet works better. It's 100 per cent effective, but also 100 per cent fatal if you manage to stick with it. This is why an optimal diet needs additional building blocks to ensure long-term viability.

Along with being efficacious and sustainable, it needs to be safe. Books touting liquid protein diets in the 1970s sold millions of copies, but the diets started killing people. Safety is about losing weight without losing your health.

Any long-term eating pattern must also be nutritionally complete, containing all essential vitamins and minerals, and finally, our chosen diet should be life-extending. In the very least, what we eat shouldn't cut our life short and

ideally should be healthy enough to improve our life spans. There's no point in losing weight if it causes you to lose it all.

After diving deep into the medical literature, I identified seventeen key ingredients to the ideal weight-loss diet and dedicated a chapter in my book *How Not to Diet* to each. The foods we eat and, in fact, our meals and entire dietary patterns should be anti-inflammatory; free from industrial pollutants; high in fibre and water; and low in high-glycemic and addictive foods, added fat and sugar, calorie density, meat, refined grains, and salt. They should also be low insulin index, friendly to our friendly gut flora, particularly satiating, and rich in fruits and vegetables as well as legumes.

We should eat real food that grows out of the ground; natural foods that come from fields, not factories; from gardens, not garbage; a diet centred on whole plant foods.

It turns out the healthiest diet also appears to be the most effective diet for weight loss. Indeed, we have experimental confirmation: a whole food, plant-based diet was found to be the single most effective weight-loss intervention ever published in the medical literature, proven in a randomized controlled trial with no portion control, no calorie counting, no exercise component – *the most effective ever*.[5]

I didn't stop there, though. I spent the second half of *How Not to Diet* on all the tools I had unearthed in my research to drive *further* weight loss for any stubborn pounds that remain.

In the first half of the book, we learned that a calorie is not necessarily a calorie. One hundred calories of chickpeas have a different impact than one hundred calories of chicken or chocolate, based on their different effects on such factors as absorption, appetite or our microbiome. In the second half, I went a step further and explained how even the exact same foods eaten differently can have different effects. It's not only *what* we eat, but *how* and *when*.

The one piece of advice that probably best sums up my recommended weight-loss boosters would be to *wall off your calories*. Animal cells are encased only in easily digestible membranes, which allow the enzymes in our gut to effortlessly liberate the calories within a steak, for example. Plant cells, on the other hand, have cell walls that are made out of fibre which acts as an indigestible physical barrier, so many of the calories remain trapped. Processed plant foods, however, such as fruit juice, sugar, refined grains, and even whole grains if they've been powdered into flour, have had their cellular structure destroyed and their cell walls cracked open, so their calories are free for the taking. When you eat structurally intact plant foods, though, you can chew all you want, but you'll still end up with calories completely encapsulated by fibre, which then blunts the glycemic impact, activates what's called the ileal brake that dials down appetite, and delivers sustenance to your friendly flora.

So, try to make sure as many of your calories – whether from protein, carbs or fat – are encased in cell walls. In other words, get as many of your calories from whole, intact plant foods.

I went into this project with the goal of creating a distillation of all the best science, but, to my delight, I discovered all sorts of exciting new tools and tricks along the way, a treasure trove of buried data, such as simple spices proven in randomized, double-blind, placebo-controlled studies to accelerate weight loss for pennies a day. With so little profit potential, it's no wonder those studies never saw the light of day. And I was even able to traverse beyond the existing evidence base to propose a new method to eliminate body fat. It can't be monetized, either, but the only profiting I care about is your health.

What appears to be the most effective weight-loss diet just so happens to be the only diet *ever* proven to reverse heart disease in the majority of patients,[6] including my own beloved grandma.

If that's all a plant-based diet could do – reverse the number one killer of men and women – shouldn't that be the default diet until proven otherwise? And the fact that it can also be effective in treating, arresting, and even reversing other leading killers, such as type 2 diabetes[7] and high blood pressure, would seem to make the case for plant-based eating simply overwhelming.

Only one diet has ever been shown to do all that: a diet centered on whole plant foods. We don't have to mortgage our health to lose weight. The single healthiest diet also appears to be the most effective diet for weight loss.

After all, permanent weight loss requires permanent dietary change. Healthier habits just need to become a way of life. And if it's going to be life-long, you want it to lead to a long life. Thankfully, the single best diet proven for weight loss may just so happen to be the safest and most inexpensive way to eat for the longest, healthiest life.

I donate to charity 100 per cent of the proceeds I get from my books – including this cookbook, *How Not to Diet*, and my best-selling *How Not to Die*, where I tackle the top fifteen killers and introduce my Daily Dozen. I don't get a single penny from my books, but I get something better – the satisfaction of helping so many people with this life-changing, lifesaving information.

I hope *The How Not to Diet Cookbook* inspires you to create delicious, healthy, sustaining meals for yourself and your family. Each recipe in this collection maximizes weight-loss potential without ever sacrificing flavour and satisfaction. And, if that weren't enough, every dish is bursting with the very foods that can play a vital role in preventing, arresting, or reversing the fifteen leading causes of death. So, get into the kitchen and cook as if your life depends on it because it very well may.

SEVENTEEN INGREDIENTS FOR AN
IDEAL WEIGHT-LOSS DIET

My original intention with *How Not to Diet*, consonant with the title, was to have chapters offering critical analysis on each of the leading popular diets, but I realized that would be like playing a game of Whac-A-Mole.

I'm a member of the *U.S. News & World Report* Best Diets expert panel, tasked with scoring dozens of trending diets based on set criteria, so I'm especially aware how many new diets pop up every year. I didn't want my book to be out of date before it even came out.

Thus, rather than taking a reactionary tack and wasting page space on Dr Quack's here-to-day-gone-tomorrow *New* Snake Oil Diet (now with added tricksy pixie dust!), I decided upon a more timeless, proactive approach: to build an optimal weight-loss diet from the ground up. On the basis of the most compelling evidence my research team and I could find, I sought to generate a list of dietary attributes and components most effectual for weight loss. The best ingredients, if you will.

I distilled this research into a list of seventeen key ingredients for an ideal weight-loss diet. These components could then be used to construct a portfolio of dietary changes to attack excess body fat on multiple fronts, as well as offer a template by which to compare any new diet that comes down the pike.

As a physician, my priority is getting (and keeping) people healthy, but when people are surveyed about their motivation for dieting, disturbingly, 'health' may come in last.[8] Dieters want results – they want weight to come off.

So, that became my challenge. If I were to construct the ideal weight-loss diet, what characteristics would it have? My research team and I dove headfirst into the nearly half-million papers published in the English-language peer-reviewed medical literature on weight management and certainly ran into some surprises on the way. What follows is my distilled list of seventeen key ingredients – dietary attributes that could be used to create the most effective eating plan for losing weight.

On the next page are the seventeen ingredients for an optimum weight-loss diet laid out in worksheet form.

In that first blank column, you can place a dietary pattern, a meal or even an individual food. Try pencilling in some of the diets you've heard about. How do they rate? How many boxes can you tick off? A paleo diet, for example, might nail the fruit-and-vegetables box but fail the legumes one.

The next time you sit down for supper, look at your meal and see how many checkmarks it earns. You can imagine how a typical fast-food meal might get a big goose egg – zero out of seventeen – whereas a healthy Mediterranean meal might hit eleven or more due to its vegetable-centric nature. A traditional Mediterranean bean-and-vegetable stew would be anti-inflammatory, low on the food chain, and high in fibre, trapped water and veggies; have a low glycemic load and insulin index; be free of habit-forming ultraprocessed foods; and could be low in added fat, sugar, meat, salt and refined grains. The beans check off legumes and microbiome-building, and soups are particularly satiating and low in calorie density. So, that one stew could potentially check off all seventeen optimal weight-loss ingredients. If you had it with bread dipped in oil, though, the meal as a whole might fail to meet the glycemic

	ANTI-INFLAMMATORY	CLEAN	↑ FIBRE	↑ WATER	↓ GLYCEMIC	↓ ADDICTIVE	↓ FAT	↓ SUGAR	↓ CALORIE DENSITY	↓ MEAT	↓ REFINED GRAINS	↓ SALT	↓ INSULIN	↑ MICROBIOME	↑ FRUITS & VEGETABLES	↑ LEGUMES	SATIATING

and insulin response criteria as well as the added fat, refined grains and sodium conditions, but it would still be better than most meals people eat.

Every meal is a new opportunity to tick as many checkmarks as you can. Imagine looking over a Chinese takeout menu. Some items, like General Tso's chicken – deep-fried meat served in a sugary sauce atop white rice – may not include any of the optimum weight-loss ingredients, whereas a dish from the vegetable section, such as broccoli with garlic sauce, might incorporate at least half of them. At a quick-service Mexican restaurant, a bean burrito bowl salad could let you tick off most of them, especially if you hold the white rice, but nothing beats the control you have at home to prepare a healthy dish without added salt, sugar, and fat.

To reverse-engineer the optimal weight-loss diet, we can figure out what constitutes the ideal meal by ranking individual foods – and the more boxes they check, the better. Most fruits and vegetables would top the list at sixteen out of seventeen. By my count, legumes, whole grains, and nuts and seeds together would hit fifteen, fourteen and thirteen, respectively, but refined grains and animal products would slip down into single digits. Ultraprocessed fatty and sugary snacks might only score one or two, and a product that's both, such as sweet-flavoured jerky, might completely flop.

Note that some of these criteria are much more important than others. For example, while the value of eating anti-inflammatory foods remains theoretical, there are multiple randomized controlled trials validating the benefits of reducing calorie density. Read through *How Not to Diet* and decide which are most convincing to you and may be easiest to fit into your daily routine.

To varying degrees, any one of these criteria alone may facilitate weight loss. Even just cutting out added sugars without making any other changes at all, for example, could cause you to lose weight.

Now imagine if you tried putting them all together.

THE DAILY DOZEN DIET

In *How Not to Die*, I compiled the healthiest of the Green Light foods – foods of plant origin from which nothing bad has been added and nothing good has been taken away – into my Daily Dozen checklist of foods I encourage people to try to fit into their daily routines. I made it into a free app, Dr Greger's Daily Dozen, available for iPhone and Android, so anyone and everyone can try to check off all the boxes every day and track their progress over time.

TOO MUCH FOOD, NOT ENOUGH CALORIES

As the feedback poured in from people using the app, two themes of complaints arose. The first was that it was just too much food. There was no way they could eat all that food in one day. In response, I explained that the Daily Dozen was aspirational, something to shoot for, just a tool to inspire people to include some of the healthiest of healthy foods into their daily diet. The vast volume of food I prescribed was on purpose.

Dr Greger's Daily Dozen

✓✓✓	BEANS
✓	BERRIES
✓✓✓	OTHER FRUITS
✓	CRUCIFEROUS VEGETABLES
✓✓	GREENS
✓✓	OTHER VEGETABLES
✓	FLAXSEEDS
✓	NUTS AND SEEDS
✓	HERBS AND SPICES
✓✓✓	WHOLE GRAINS
✓✓✓✓	BEVERAGES
✓	EXERCISE

Here is the Daily Dozen and the number of servings I recommend for each one. For years, I had this list on a little dry-erase board on our refrigerator. Feel free to cut this one out (or make your own copy) and do the same. It's also useful to take with you when you go shopping to guide you through your healthiest choices. And remember, it's just about doing your best. There are times, especially when I am travelling, that I only hit a quarter of my goals. When that happens, I just try to make up for it the next day. The same goes for you: If one day you only get a few of these foods into your diet, the next day, do your best to get more!

I was hoping that by telling people to eat so much healthy stuff, it would naturally crowd out some of the less healthy stuff. After checking off all twenty-four servings in the Daily Dozen, there's only so much room left for a pepperoni pizza.

Ironically, the second major complaint we got is that it doesn't have enough calories. I had to explain that the Daily Dozen just represented the minimum I encourage people to eat, not the maximum, and that, certainly, training athletes requiring thousands more calories would have to eat much more. This all got me thinking, though. *Too much food but too few calories?* Sounds like the perfect weight-loss diet!

The Daily Dozen is by definition all Green Light foods, all whole plant foods, so that right there bakes in all seventeen of the ideal weight-loss diet ingredients listed on page xii. What about the calorie count? A systematic review of successful weight-loss strategies concluded that given the metabolic slowing and increased appetite that accompanies weight loss, to achieve significant weight loss, calorie counts may need to drop as low as 1,200 calories a day for women and 1,500 calories a day for men.[9] I set up a spreadsheet and tried a bunch of common foods in each of the categories, and what do you know: the Daily Dozen averages about 1,200 calories, with the higher-calorie food choices nailing 1,500 calories.

GREEN LIGHT FOR WEIGHT LOSS

How is my Green Light category in *How Not to Die* different from my recommendation in *How Not to Diet* to wall off your calories, to ensure your protein, carbs, and fat are trapped within cell walls? After all, only plants have cell walls. (Animals are made up of cells with fluid membranes, requiring bones to hold them up, whereas plants have rigid cell walls made out of fibre.) So, isn't walling off calories the same as choosing whole plant foods? The difference becomes apparent with examples of formless foods, such as powdered whole grains. Imagine a whole-grain wheat cereal with one ingredient: 100% whole wheat. Or almond butter with one ingredient: almonds. Green Light, right? Plant foods from which nothing bad has been added and nothing good has been taken away. But now we know something good has been taken away: the structure.

Eating whole grains is good, but eating whole-grain kernels is better. Former Harvard nutrition chair Walter Willett has argued that the term *whole grain* should probably be reserved for only whole, intact grain kernels.[10] So, eat the wholiest of grains: intact grains, also known as groats.

Take oats, for example. They're found out in the fields as oat groats and then have their inedible outer husks removed during processing.[11] Groats can then be sliced into two to four pieces to make steel-cut (also known as pinhead or Irish) oats, coarsely ground into Scottish oatmeal, or steamed and flattened into 'old-fashioned' rolled oats.[12] Quick-cooking oats are just old-fashioned oats rolled even thinner, and instant oats are steamed longer and rolled even more thinly.[13] Then, at the bottom of the list, the most processed would be powdered oats, which you might find in oat-based breakfast cereals. Instead of buying boxed breakfast cereals, make oatmeal out of whole, intact oats. They're gr-r-oat!

With all the new data on the importance of food form, I'm starting to sour on flour, so I advise not living by bread alone. The new structure created by the pasta-making process can mediate these effects, though, so you don't have to say *basta* to pasta.

OPTIMIZING THE DAILY DOZEN FOR WEIGHT LOSS

A typical Green Light foods breakfast that would check off a few of the Daily Dozen boxes would be a big bowl of oatmeal sweetened with raisins. On the basis of what we learned in the Low in Calorie Density, High in Water-Rich Foods, Eating Rate, and Wall Off Your Calories sections of *How Not to Diet*, though, we could optimize that meal for weight loss by making the oatmeal from steel-cut or whole groats rather than rolled or instant, cooking it thick, and switching the dried fruit for fresh – for example, swapping in strawberries for the raisins. If we did want to use dried, as we learned in the Amping AMPK and Inflammation Quenchers sections, barberries or gojis might be a better choice.

Similarly, when choosing vegetables, we can steer toward aboveground veggies highest on the water scale. Peppers have that nicotine edge I described in Amping AMPK, and uncooked vegetables in general offer more orosensory stimulation. If you want to go underground, on the basis of what we learned about glycemic load, sweet potatoes would be preferable to white. We certainly want to mix it up, though, to take advantage of our built-in striving for variety, and since vegetables represent the healthiest class of foods with the fewest calories, we should aim to eat them earlier in the meal.

In the Appetite Suppression section, we learned yet another reason to include ground flaxseeds in our daily diet. Nuts are a great complement to greens to boost the absorption of fat-soluble nutrients, but, ideally, they should be eaten raw and whole or coarsely chopped rather than blended into butters. This is not to say something like almond butter or tahini is unhealthy by any stretch, but for weight-loss acceleration, structurally intact nuts and seeds would be better.

TWENTY-ONE TWEAKS TO ACCELERATE WEIGHT LOSS

Offering maximum nutrition with minimum calories, a diet centered on whole, healthy plant foods is the best form of girth control. Whole food, plant-based nutrition best checks off the criteria for the optimal slimming diet. It's the tried-and-true recipe with the most ideal weight-loss diet ingredients – so why wasn't that the end of *How Not to Diet*?

Just eating healthfully enough should do it. Obese individuals randomized to eat plant-based at home lose nearly a cubic inch of deep visceral belly fat a week.[14] Start packing your diet with real food that grows out of the ground, and the pounds should come off naturally, taking you down toward your ideal weight. The average person eating completely plant-based has a body mass index (BMI) down around the perfect range,[15] but there is a bell curve. Even if the average is on target, some people naturally fall to either side, so I wanted to offer an array of tools that can drive or boost further weight loss for any stubborn pounds that remain.

That was the reason all the chapters in *How Not to Die* on the leading killer diseases were longer than just the three words: eat more plants. Yes, those who go all in should end up with perfect blood pressure and perfect cholesterol levels on average, for example, but if you're doing everything right and your numbers are still off, I wanted to go through all the dietary tweaks you could use to optimize your condition. That way, you could create a portfolio of specific foods to help with each specific condition. I wanted to do the same thing with *How Not to Diet*.

My hope is to give you an arsenal of weapons in your fight against fat.

The average, purely plant-based person has an ideal BMI, which greatly incentivizes sticking with that way of eating, but if that's not where you end up or if you just want to get there quicker, are there specific plants that have an edge? And not some tabloid-y, fat-busting 'breakthrough' extrapolated from test-tube data or mouse models but from actual randomized, controlled, clinical trials showing objective outcomes?

Yes, there are specific foods shown in interventional studies to cause you to burn more fat, suppress your appetite, rev up your metabolism, block the absorption of calories and effectively take away even more calories than they provide. What's more, the context in which we eat matters, too. The same number of calories eaten at a different time of the day, in a different meal distribution or after different amounts of sleep can translate into different amounts of body fat.

Distinct forms of the exact same foods can be distinctly fattening. Combining certain foods together can have a different effect from eating them apart.

What we eat matters most, but how we eat and when can also make a difference. Even the exact same foods eaten differently can have different effects.

Importantly, these tricks and tweaks serve to supplement a healthy, lifelong eating pattern, not replace it. Eliminating obesity requires treating the cause, the underlying diet, but my weight-loss boosters are for those who want all the extra help they can get.

A HEFTIER DAILY DOZEN APP

My free Dr Greger's Daily Dozen app released soon after publication of *How Not to Die* had become so popular that I decided to completely revamp it with new features for *How Not to Diet*. I incorporated all these tweaks to the Daily Dozen to optimize it for weight control. Now, you can not only track your progress, graphing your momentum day to day and month to month to see how well you're nailing each of the Daily Dozen, but since so many seemed to really appreciate having a list of reminders to check off throughout the day, I added an entirely new checklist to capture the weight-loss boosters I documented in *How Not to Diet*. With the new, expanded version of the app, you can track your weight and make a game out of how many of the new fat-busting boosters you can squeeze in every day, along with your Daily Dozen checkboxes.

Dr Greger's 21 Tweaks

AT EACH MEAL

√√√ PRELOAD WITH WATER

√√√ PRELOAD WITH 'NEGATIVE CALORIE' FOODS

√√√ INCORPORATE VINEGAR (2 tsp with each meal)

√√√ ENJOY UNDISTRACTED MEALS

√√√ FOLLOW THE 20-MINUTE RULE

EVERY DAY

TAKE YOUR DAILY DOSES

√ NIGELLA SEEDS (¼ tsp)

√ GARLIC POWDER (¼ tsp)

√ GROUND GINGER (1 tsp) or CAYENNE PEPPER (½ tsp)

√ NUTRITIONAL YEAST (2 tsp)

√ CUMIN (½ tsp with lunch and dinner)

√ GREEN TEA (3 cups tea)

√ STAY HYDRATED

√ DEFLOUR YOUR DIET

√ FRONT-LOAD CALORIES

√ TIME-RESTRICT YOUR EATING

√ OPTIMIZE EXCERCISE TIMING

√√ WEIGH YOURSELF TWICE A DAY

√√√ COMPLETE YOUR IMPLEMENTATION INTENTIONS

EVERY NIGHT

√ FAST AFTER 7:00 PM

√ GET SUFFICIENT SLEEP

√ EXPERIMENT WITH MILD TRENDELENBURG

BOXES OF TRICKS

Some of the weight-loss boosters are automatically taken care of with the Daily Dozen. For example, fat-blocking thylakoids and calcium are covered with my recommendation to eat lots of low-oxalate greens. But for the others, I developed my Twenty-One Tweaks, practical takeaways from the boosters collected into one simple list.

You may have noticed that not all the strategies I covered in part 4 of *How Not to Diet* are included in the list. Some only apply to certain individuals. For example, asking people to get into the NEAT habit of using steppers, fidget bars, or bouncing their knees during prolonged sitting may only apply to those with desk jobs. Other accelerants may be too risky for general consumption. For example, while the 25:5 modified fasting shows promise, you probably shouldn't drop below 1,000 calories a day for more than twenty-four hours without medical supervision.[16] Finally, there are options that show theoretical promise but haven't been sufficiently vetted in clinical trials, such as pistachios for circadian synchronization or mixing peppermint oil into hand lotion to facilitate brown adipose tissue (BAT) activation.

So, here's the list of strategies that made the cut – broadly applicable, relatively safe, and evidence based. See how many of these easily actionable tweaks you can incorporate into your daily routine.

AT EACH MEAL

PRELOAD WITH WATER
Time a metabolism-boosting 2 glasses (about 500ml) of cool or cold unflavoured water before each meal to take advantage of its preload benefits.

PRELOAD WITH 'NEGATIVE CALORIE' FOODS
As the first course, start each meal with an apple or a Green Light soup or salad containing fewer than 100 calories per cup (around 250ml or 200g, depending on ingredients). Soups and salads that fit this criterion are marked throughout the cookbook.

INCORPORATE VINEGAR (2 TEASPOONS WITH EACH MEAL)
Never drink vinegar straight. Instead, flavour meals or dress a side salad with any of the sweet or savoury vinegars out there. If you want to drink it, make sure to mix it in a glass of water, and afterwards, be sure to rinse your mouth out with water to protect your tooth enamel.

ENJOY UNDISTRACTED MEALS
Don't eat while watching TV or playing on your phone. Give yourself a check for each meal you're able to eat without distraction.

FOLLOW THE TWENTY-MINUTE RULE
Whether through increasing viscosity or the number of chews or decreasing bite size and eating rate, dozens of studies have demonstrated that no matter how we boost the amount of time food is in our mouths, it can result in lower caloric intake. So, extend meal duration to at least twenty minutes to allow your natural satiety signals to take full effect. How? By choosing foods that take longer to eat and eating them in a way that prolongs the time they stay in your mouth. Think bulkier, harder, chewier foods in smaller, well-chewed bites.

EVERY DAY

TAKE YOUR DAILY DOSES

Nigella Seeds (*Nigella sativa*) (¼ teaspoon) As noted in the Appetite Suppression section of *How Not to Diet*, a systematic review and meta-analysis of randomized, controlled weight-loss trials found that about ¼ teaspoon of nigella seed powder every day appears to reduce body mass index within a span of a couple of months.

Garlic Powder (¼ teaspoon) Randomized, double-blind, placebo-controlled studies have found that as little as a daily ¼ teaspoon of garlic powder can reduce body fat at a cost of a few pence a day.

Ground Ginger (1 teaspoon) or Cayenne (½ teaspoon) Randomized controlled trials have found that ¼ to 1½ teaspoons a day of ground ginger significantly decreased body weight for just pennies a day. It can be as easy as stirring the ground spice into a cup of hot water. Ginger may work better in the morning than evening, and consider chai tea as a tasty way to combine the green tea and ginger tricks into a single beverage.

Alternately, for BAT activation, you can add one raw jalapeño pepper or ½ teaspoon of red pepper powder (or, presumably, crushed red pepper flakes) into your daily diet. To help beat the heat, you can very thinly slice or finely chop the jalapeño to reduce its bite to little prickles, or mix the red pepper into soup or the whole food vegetable smoothie featured in one of my cooking videos on NutritionFacts.org.[17]

Nutritional Yeast (2 teaspoons) Two teaspoons of baker's, brewer's, or nutritional yeast contain roughly the amount of beta 1,3/1,6 glucans found in randomized, double-blind, placebo-controlled clinical trials to facilitate weight loss.

Cumin (*Cuminum cyminum*) (½ teaspoon with lunch and dinner) Overweight women randomized to add ½ teaspoon of ground cumin to each lunch and dinner beat the control group by four more pounds and an extra inch off their waist. There is also evidence to support the use of the spice saffron, but a pinch a day would cost a lot, whereas a teaspoon of cumin costs very little.

Green Tea (3 cups) Drink 3 cups a day between meals (waiting at least an hour after a meal so as to not interfere with iron absorption). During meals, drink water, black coffee or hibiscus tea mixed 6:1 with lemon verbena, but never exceed 3 cups of fluid per hour. This is important, given my water preloading advice.

Take advantage of the reinforcing effect of caffeine by drinking your green tea along with something healthy you wish you liked more, but don't consume large amounts of caffeine within six hours of bedtime. Taking your tea without sweetener is best, but if you typically sweeten your tea with honey or sugar, try yacón syrup instead.

STAY HYDRATED

Check this box if your urine never appears darker than a pale yellow. Note that if you're eating riboflavin-fortified foods (such as nutritional yeast), then base this instead on getting 9 cups of unsweetened beverages a day for women (which would be taken care of by the green tea and water preloading recommendations) or 13 cups a day for men. If you have heart or kidney issues, don't increase fluid intake at all without first talking with your doctor. Remember, diet soda may be calorie free, but it's not consequence free, as we learned in the Low in Added Sugar section of *How Not to Diet*.

DEFLOUR YOUR DIET

Check this box every day your whole-grain servings are in the form of intact grains. The powdering of even 100% whole grains robs our microbiome of the starch that would otherwise be ferried down to our colon enclosed in unbroken cell walls.

FRONT-LOAD YOUR CALORIES

There are metabolic benefits to distributing more calories to earlier in the day, so make breakfast (ideally) or lunch your largest meal of the day in true king/prince/pauper style.

TIME-RESTRICT YOUR EATING

Confine eating to a daily window of time of your choosing under twelve hours in length that you can stick to consistently, seven days a week. Given the circadian benefits of reducing evening food intake, the window should end before 7:00 p.m.

OPTIMIZE EXERCISE TIMING

The Daily Dozen's recommendation for optimum exercise duration for longevity is ninety minutes of moderately intense activity a day, which is also the optimum exercise duration for weight loss. Anytime is good, and the more the better, but there may be an advantage to exercising in a fasted state, at least six hours after your last meal. Typically, this would mean before breakfast, but if you timed it right, you could exercise midday before a late lunch or, if lunch is eaten early enough, before dinner. This is the timing for nondiabetics.

Diabetics and prediabetics should instead start exercising thirty minutes after the start of a meal and ideally go for at least an hour to completely straddle the blood sugar peak. If you had to choose a single meal to exercise after, it would be dinner, due to the circadian rhythm of blood sugar control that wanes throughout the day. Ideally, though, breakfast would be the largest meal of the day, and you'd exercise after that – or, even better, after every meal.

WEIGH YOURSELF TWICE A DAY

Regular self-weighing is considered crucial for long-term weight control, but there is insufficient evidence to support a specific frequency of weighing. My recommendation is based on the one study that found that twice daily – upon waking and right before bed – appeared superior to once a day (about 6 versus 2 pounds of weight loss over 12 weeks).

COMPLETE YOUR IMPLEMENTATION INTENTIONS

Every two months, create three new implementation intentions – 'if X, then Y' plans to perform a particular behavior in a specific context – and check each one of them off as you complete them every day.

EVERY NIGHT

FAST AFTER 7:00 P.M.

Because of our circadian rhythm, food eaten at night is more fattening than the exact same food eaten earlier in the day, so fast every night for at least twelve hours starting before 7:00 p.m. The fewer calories after sundown, the better.

GET SUFFICIENT SLEEP

Check this box if you get at least seven hours of sleep at your regular bedtime.

EXPERIMENT WITH MILD TRENDELENBURG

Try spending at least four hours a night lying with your body tilted head-down 6 degrees by elevating the posts at the foot of your bed by 20 cm (or by 25 cm if your bed is extra long). Be extremely careful when you get out of bed, as this may cause orthostatic intolerance, even if you're young and healthy – meaning if you get up too fast, you can feel dizzy, faint or light-headed and could fall and hurt yourself. So, get up slowly. Drinking a large glass of cold water (around 500ml) thirty minutes before rising may also help prevent this potentially hazardous side effect.

IMPORTANT: Do not try this at home at all if you have any heart or lung issues, acid reflux, or problems with your brain (e.g., head trauma) or eyes (even a family history of glaucoma disqualifies you). Also do not try this until you ask your doctor whether he or she thinks it's safe for you to sleep in mild Trendelenburg.

TICK ALL THE RIGHT BOXES

Between the twenty-four checkoffs in the Daily Dozen and the thirty-four new checkoffs in the Tweaks, you may feel a bit overwhelmed, but it's easy to knock off a bunch at a time. For example, starting a meal with a tomato salad sprinkled with some nigella seeds, garlic powder and balsamic vinegar hits five boxes right there, including the 'Preload with "Negative Calorie" Foods' tweak and the Daily Dozen box for 'Other Vegetables'. And if that was one of your implementation intentions, make that six! Ten per cent of your boxes nailed with a single appetizer.

Of course, you don't have to hit all the booster boxes every day. You don't even have to hit any. A healthy diet, as encapsulated by the Daily Dozen, should be all you need to lose as much weight as you want, but the more of these extra tweaks you can hit, the more successful you may be.

The How Not to Diet Cookbook fits as many of these combinations together into delicious recipes and hearty meal plans, and please feel free to download the free, updated Dr Greger's Daily Dozen app on your Android or iPhone. Start experimenting with a few of the Twenty-One Tweaks and see which ones work for you. My goal is to just provide you with the broadest palette of tools to choose from.

Remember, it's not what you eat today that matters, or tomorrow, or next week, but rather what you eat over the next months, years, and decades, so you have to find lifestyle changes that fit into your lifestyle.

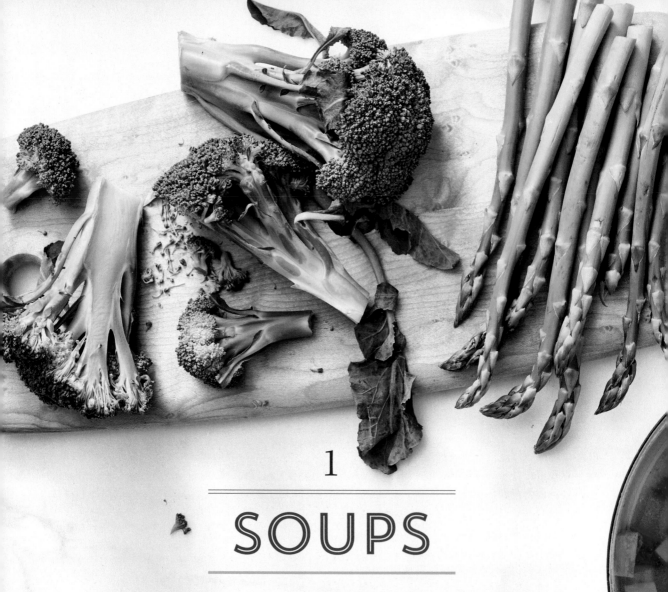

1

SOUPS

Filling, satisfying, comforting. Soup is all of these and even more when it comes to weight loss. If you give people a casserole for lunch, they eat the same amount whether or not they're also given a glass of water, about 400 calories' worth. But if that same casserole and that same water are blended into a soup, they only eat 300 calories' worth before feeling full.[18] Blended together, the same meal components served as a soup left people feeling significantly fuller even three hours later.[19] What's so special about soup? Time. Eating more slowly may reduce caloric intake. What's more, soup consumers tend to have a slimmer waist and lower body weight, and also tend to exhibit other healthy eating behaviours, such as eating more greens and beans.[20]

I love every one of the soups featured in this cookbook, but what I love even more is how they make me feel, inside and out.

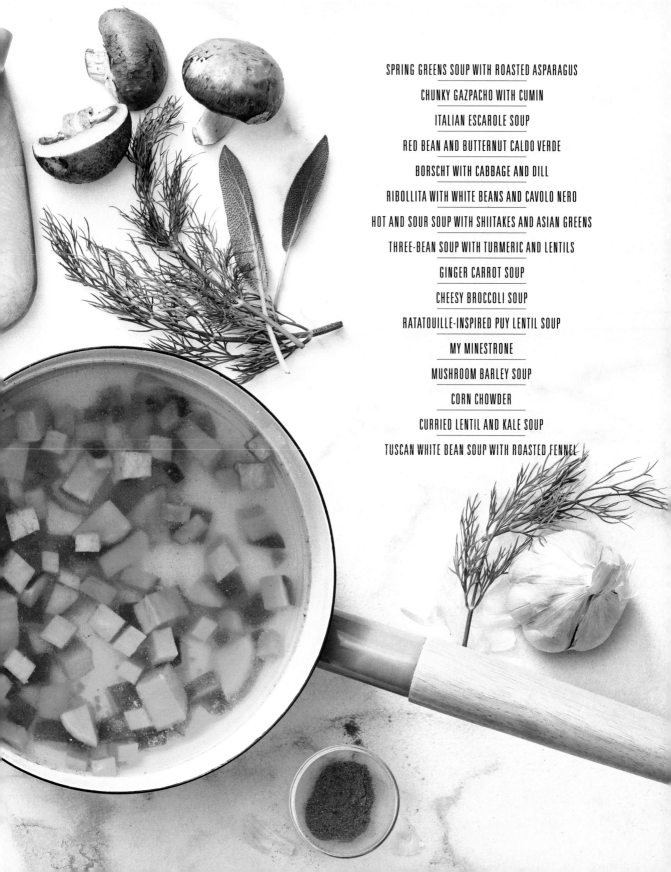

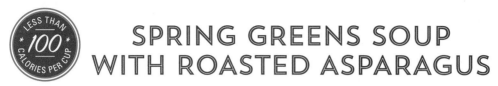

SPRING GREENS SOUP WITH ROASTED ASPARAGUS

MAKES: *4 servings*   DIFFICULTY: *Easy*

This bright and comforting soup is packed with fresh greens, peas and roasted asparagus. Enjoy it hot, warm or chilled.

8 ounces/225g thin asparagus, trimmed and cut into 1½-inch (4cm) pieces (reserve the tips)

1 onion, chopped

2 teaspoons finely chopped garlic

6 cups/1.5 litres Light Vegetable Broth (page 214)

6 cups/150g coarsely chopped spinach or chard

2 cups/50g coarsely chopped rocket, watercress or mustard greens

1 cup/150g fresh or thawed frozen peas

3 spring onions, coarsely chopped

1 tablespoon nutritional yeast

1 teaspoon white miso paste

Ground black pepper

1 tablespoon fresh lemon juice

1 tablespoon coarsely ground nigella seeds

Preheat the oven to 200°C/400°F/gas mark 6. Line a rimmed roasting tin with a silicone mat or baking parchment.

Arrange all of the cut asparagus in the prepared roasting tin in a single layer, but keep the tips separate from the rest of the asparagus. Roast in the oven until tender and the edges begin to brown, about 15 minutes. Remove from the oven and set aside, again keeping the tips separate.

Heat ¼ cup/60ml of water in a large saucepan over medium heat. Add the onion and cook until softened, about 5 minutes. Add the garlic and cook, stirring, for another minute. Add the Light Vegetable Broth and bring to the boil. Lower the heat to a simmer and cook for 7 minutes. Remove the pot from the heat. Stir in the spinach, rocket, peas and spring onions and cook until the greens are wilted and tender from the hot broth, about 2 minutes. Stir in the roasted asparagus (except the tips), nutritional yeast, miso paste and black pepper to taste.

Working in batches, transfer the soup to a high-powered blender and blend until smooth. Return the soup to the pot and heat, if desired. Stir in the lemon juice and then taste and adjust the seasonings, if needed. Ladle the soup into bowls and top with the asparagus tips and nigella seeds.

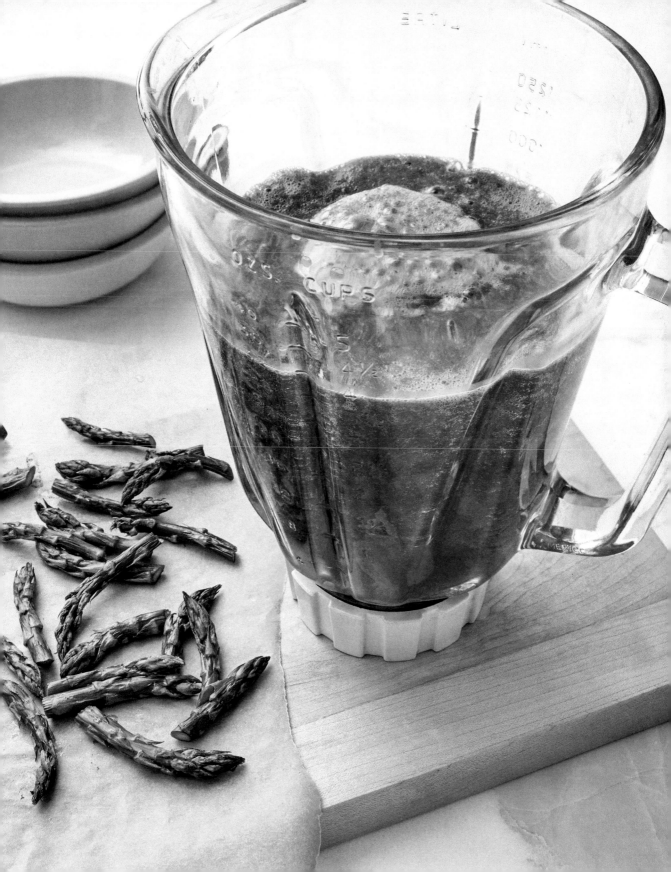

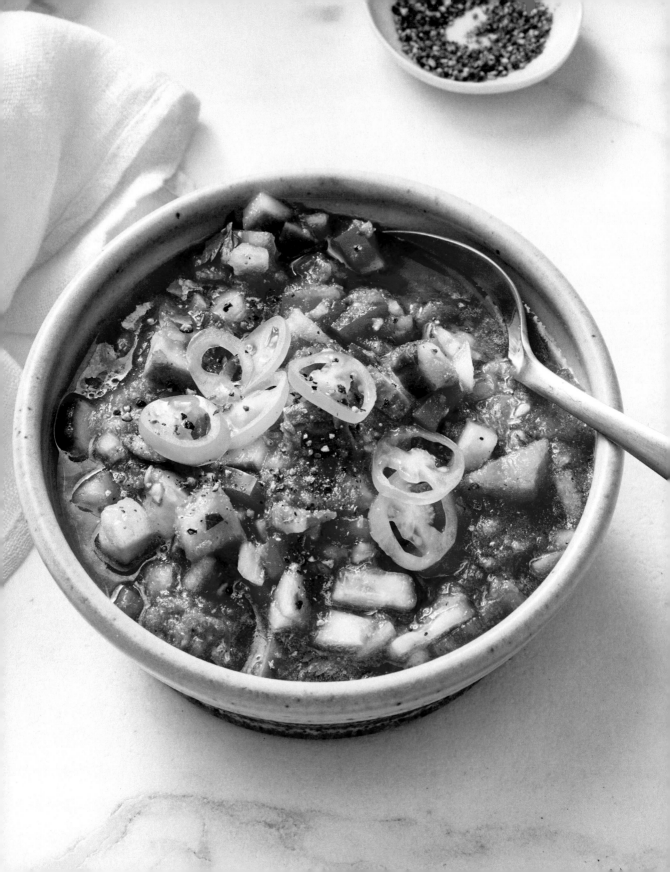

CHUNKY GAZPACHO
WITH CUMIN

MAKES: *4 servings*   DIFFICULTY: *Easy*

Cumin lovers take note: with cumin featured in this soup twice, this soup is for you.

2 mini cucumbers, peeled and chopped

1 red pepper, de-seeded and chopped

2½ pounds/1.1kg ripe tomatoes, cored and chopped

⅓ cup/50g chopped onion

1 garlic clove, chopped

3 tablespoons finely chopped fresh parsley

2½ tablespoons sherry vinegar or red wine vinegar

Super-Charged Spice Blend (page 211)

½ teaspoon ground cumin

¼ teaspoon ground black pepper

1 teaspoon Salt-Free Hot Sauce (page 216; optional)

2 tablespoons finely chopped spring onion

2 tablespoons chopped fresh coriander or basil

6 firm yellow cherry tomatoes, thinly sliced (optional)

1 teaspoon coarsely ground nigella seeds

In a large bowl, combine 1 chopped cucumber, half of the chopped pepper, half of the chopped tomatoes and the chopped onion. Set aside.

In a blender or food processor, combine the garlic with the remaining cucumber, remaining chopped pepper and remaining chopped tomatoes and process until smooth. Pour the pureed vegetables into the same bowl as the chopped vegetables. Add the parsley, vinegar, Super-Charged Spice Blend to taste, cumin, black pepper and Salt-Free Hot Sauce (if using).

Cover the bowl and refrigerate for at least 2 hours, preferably overnight, to chill and allow the flavours to develop.

Stir in the spring onion and coriander. Taste and adjust the seasonings, if needed. Serve the soup chilled, garnished with the yellow tomato slices (if using) and sprinkled with the nigella seeds.

ITALIAN ESCAROLE SOUP

MAKES: *4 servings*   DIFFICULTY: *Easy*

A member of the chicory family, escarole is a hearty bitter green widely used in Italian cooking and is frequently paired with cannellini beans. Endive or chicory would also taste good.

4 garlic cloves, finely chopped

2 medium heads escarole, chopped

6 cups/1.5 litres Light Vegetable Broth (page 214)

3 cups/525g cooked* or 2 (400g) BPA-free tins or Tetra Paks** salt-free cannellini beans, drained and rinsed

2 teaspoons Dr Greger's Special Spice Blend (page 212), or to taste

½ teaspoon dried oregano

½ teaspoon garlic powder

½ teaspoon onion powder

¼ teaspoon red pepper flakes, or to taste

1 tablespoon nutritional yeast

Ground black pepper

Heat ¼ cup/60ml water in a large pot over medium heat. Add the garlic and cook until fragrant, about 30 seconds. Add the escarole and cook, stirring, until wilted, about 4 minutes. Pour in the Light Vegetable Broth. Add the beans, Dr Greger's Special Spice Blend, oregano, garlic powder, onion powder, red pepper flakes, nutritional yeast and black pepper to taste. Cover and simmer until the escarole is tender and the soup is heated through, about 30 minutes.

*Turn to the Legumes and Grains Cooking Charts *on pages 218–221 for instruction, if needed.*

**Tetra Pak is a type of aseptic packaging, free from contamination from bacteria and other microorganisms, so the food has a very long shelf life.*

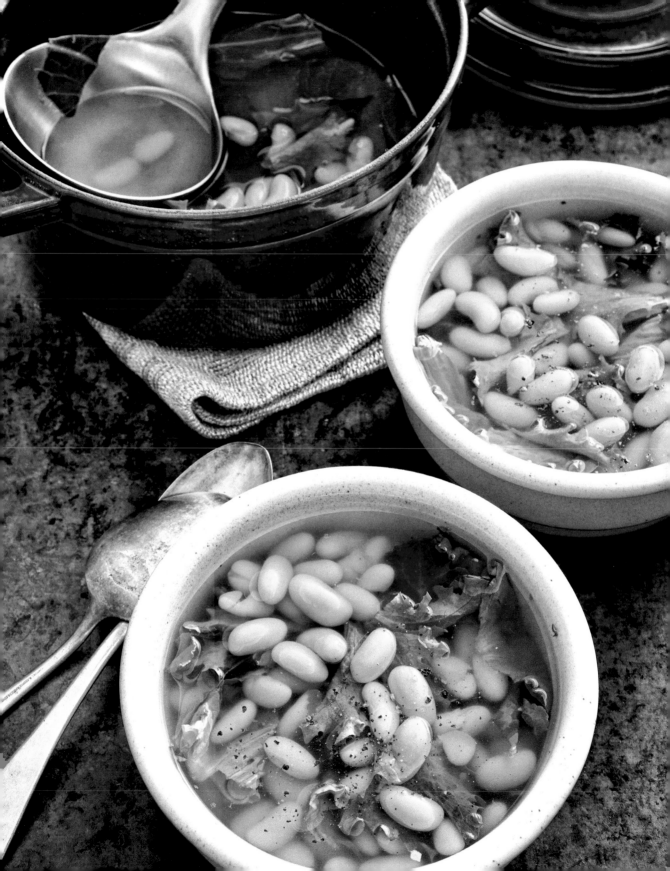

RED BEAN AND BUTTERNUT CALDO VERDE

MAKES: *4 servings*   DIFFICULTY: *Easy*

The traditional Portuguese soup is made with dark greens, potatoes and sliced sausage, but this elevated, healthier version keeps the greens while swapping in butternut squash for potatoes (though you can add potatoes, too, if you'd like*) and replaces the sausage with red kidney beans.

1 red onion, chopped

4 garlic cloves, finely chopped

1 butternut squash, halved, de-seeded and cut into ½-inch (1cm) dice (about 3½ cups/490g)

½ teaspoon dried oregano

¼ teaspoon red pepper flakes, or to taste

2 bay leaves

6 cups/1.5 litres Light Vegetable Broth (page 214)

6 cups/220g chopped fresh kale, collards or other dark greens

1½ cups/265g cooked** or 1 (400g) BPA-free tin or Tetra Pak salt-free red kidney beans, drained and rinsed

Super-Charged Spice Blend (page 211)

1 teaspoon white miso paste

3 tablespoons nutritional yeast

2 tablespoons chopped fresh parsley

Heat ¼ cup/60ml water in a large pot over medium heat. Add the onion, garlic, squash, oregano, red pepper flakes and bay leaves. Cover and cook for 5 minutes. Stir in the Light Vegetable Broth and bring to the boil. Lower the heat to a simmer and cook, partially covered, until the vegetables are just tender, about 20 minutes. Stir in the kale, kidney beans and Super-Charged Spice Blend to taste and cook for 10 minutes longer.

In a small bowl, combine the miso paste with about ¼ cup/60ml of the hot broth, stirring to blend. Pour the miso mixture into the soup and remove and discard the bay leaves. Stir in the nutritional yeast and parsley. Taste and adjust the seasoning, if needed. Serve hot.

I left white potatoes out of my How Not to Die Cookbook *because there are healthier choices, such as sweet potatoes, but, as I noted in* How Not to Diet, *plain potatoes rank as one of the most satiating foods ever tested, so they made the cut for this collection of recipes.*

**Turn to the* Legumes and Grains Cooking Charts *on pages 218–221 for instruction, if needed.*

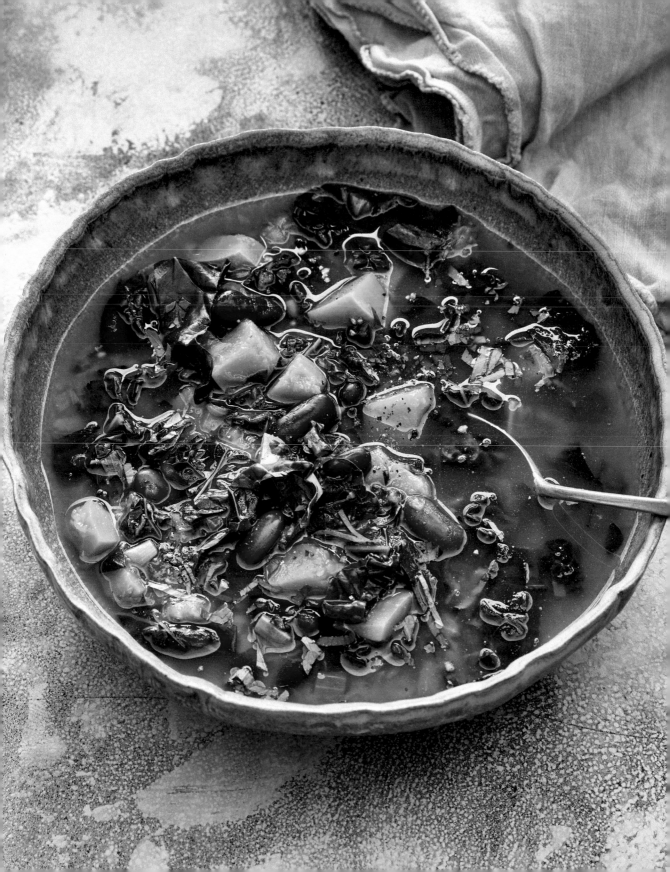

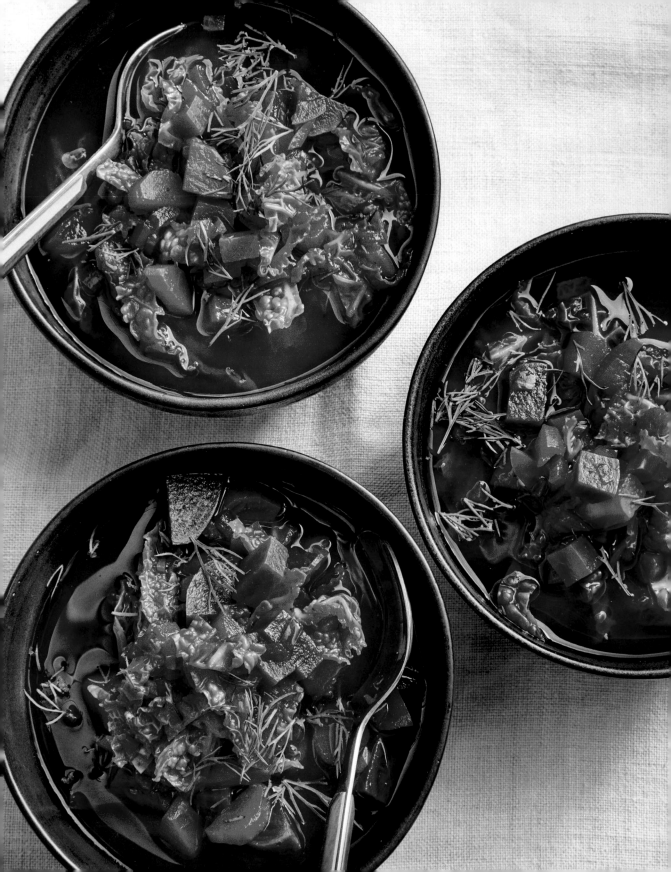

BORSCHT WITH CABBAGE AND DILL

MAKES: *4 servings*   **DIFFICULTY:** *Easy*

Beetroot may be the star of this soup, but there are a lot of supporting players, from cabbage to parsnips, and a seasoning of fresh dill and a splash of vinegar brighten the flavour.

1 red onion, chopped

2 garlic cloves, finely chopped

1 celery stalk, chopped

1 parsnip, chopped

1 carrot, chopped

3 beetroot, peeled and chopped

2 tablespoons salt-free tomato puree

6 cups/1.5 litres Light Vegetable Broth (page 214)

4 cups/400g shredded savoy cabbage

1 teaspoon dried marjoram

1 bay leaf

2 teaspoons Dr Greger's Special Spice Blend (page 212), or to taste

½ teaspoon ground black pepper

¼ cup/4 tablespoons finely chopped fresh dill

1 to 2 tablespoons red wine vinegar, or to taste

Heat ¼ cup/60ml water in a large pot over medium heat. Add the onion and garlic. Cook, stirring frequently, until the onion is softened, about 5 minutes. Add the celery, parsnip, carrot and beetroot. Cover and cook over a low heat, stirring occasionally, until the vegetables are slightly tender, about 7 minutes.

Add the tomato puree, Light Vegetable Broth, cabbage, marjoram, bay leaf, Dr Greger's Special Spice Blend and black pepper. Bring the soup to the boil, then lower the heat to a simmer, partially cover and cook for 30 minutes, or until the vegetables are completely tender.

Remove and discard the bay leaf and stir in the dill and red wine vinegar. Taste and adjust the seasonings, if needed.

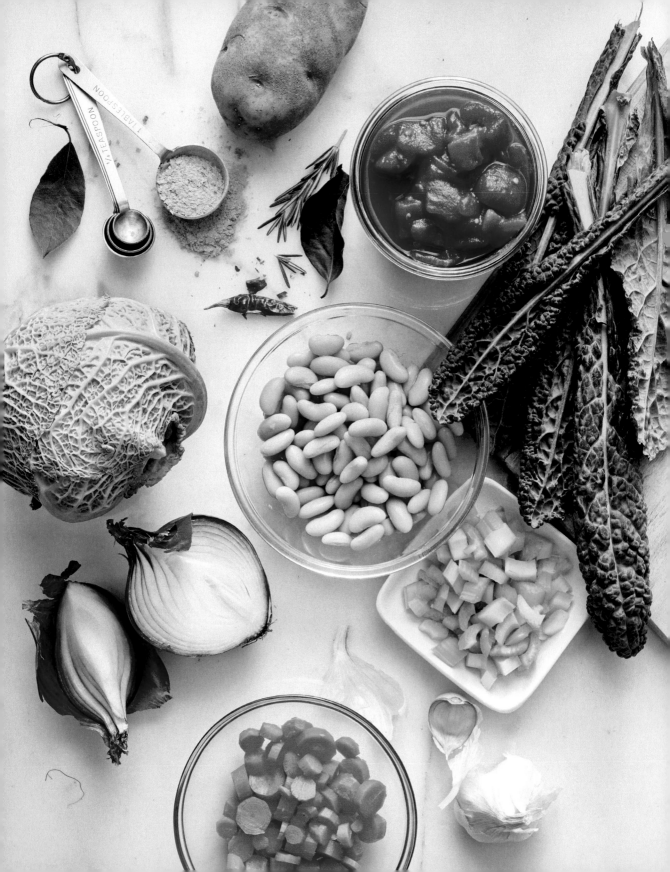

RIBOLLITA WITH WHITE BEANS AND CAVOLO NERO

MAKES: *6 servings*   DIFFICULTY: *Easy*

Ribollita is an Italian peasant soup that, like most soups, tastes even better when reheated and served the next day, as the flavours are allowed to develop even more – hence the name *ribollita*, which means 'reboiled'. Traditional ribollita contains Parmesan and chunks of crusty Italian bread, but this cleaner, more modern version skips the cheese and bread in favour of superstars cavolo nero and cabbage. This soup is delicious no matter when you enjoy it, but if you have time, try to prepare it a day before you plan to serve it so it's truly a ribollita, a 'reboiled' peasant soup.

1 large red onion, chopped

4 garlic cloves, finely chopped

2 carrots, chopped

6 cups/1.5 litres Light Vegetable Broth (page 214)

2 celery stalks, chopped

2 floury potatoes, diced

1 head savoy cabbage, chopped

1 bunch cavolo nero, chopped

2 (400g) BPA-free tins or Tetra Paks salt-free chopped tomatoes, undrained

3 cups/525g cooked* or 2 (400g) BPA-free tins or Tetra Paks salt-free cannellini beans, drained and rinsed

¼ to ½ teaspoon red pepper flakes

1 sprig rosemary

1 bay leaf

3 tablespoons nutritional yeast

Heat ¼ cup/60ml water in a large pot over a medium heat. Add the onion, garlic and carrots. Cover and cook, stirring occasionally, until the vegetables have softened, about 5 minutes. Add the Light Vegetable Broth, celery, potatoes, cabbage, cavolo nero, tomatoes, beans, red pepper flakes, rosemary sprig and bay leaf. Bring to the boil, then lower the heat to a simmer, and continue to cook until the vegetables are very soft, about 45 minutes. Remove and discard the rosemary sprig and bay leaf, and stir in the nutritional yeast. Serve hot.

*Turn to the Legumes and Grains Cooking Charts *on pages 218–221 for instruction, if needed.*

THE BENEFITS OF KALE AND CABBAGE FOR CHOLESTEROL

Increased fruit and vegetable consumption can help reduce risk of heart disease and strokes, partly due to their antioxidants preventing the oxidation of bad LDL cholesterol.[21] Study subjects ate kale and cabbage every day for two weeks and got increased antioxidant capacity of their blood and significant reductions of total cholesterol, LDL cholesterol, blood sugar levels, and oxidized LDL.[22]

HOT AND SOUR SOUP WITH SHIITAKES AND ASIAN GREENS

MAKES: *4 servings*   DIFFICULTY: *Easy*

This soup is easily customizable to please your palate. If you don't like spicy food, feel free to cut back on the hot chillies or even skip them altogether, for instance. And if you prefer as heartier soup, add some cooked whole grains or 100% buckwheat noodles just before serving.

6 cups/1.5 litres Light Vegetable Broth (page 214)

1 (4-inch/10cm) piece lemongrass, crushed

2 (¼-inch/1cm) slices fresh ginger

1 garlic clove, crushed

4 cups/400g thinly sliced bok choy, napa cabbage or other Asian greens

3 cups/225g sliced shiitake mushroom caps

2 shallots, cut lengthways into thin slivers

1 or 2 serrano or other small hot chillies, de-seeded and thinly sliced

1 cup/110g grated carrot

2 cups/300g cherry tomatoes, quartered

3 spring onions, chopped

2 tablespoons apple cider vinegar

2 teaspoons Dr Greger's Special Spice Blend (page 212), or to taste

¼ cup/4 tablespoons chopped fresh coriander or Thai basil

In a large pot, combine the Light Vegetable Broth, lemongrass, ginger and garlic. Bring to the boil, then lower the heat to low, cover and simmer for 20 minutes. Strain the broth through a sieve and discard the aromatics.

Return the broth to the large pot and bring to the boil. Add the bok choy, mushrooms, shallots, chillies and carrot. Lower the heat to low and cook for 5 minutes. Stir in the tomatoes, spring onions, apple cider vinegar and Dr Greger's Special Spice Blend. Simmer until hot, about 3 minutes. Taste and adjust the seasonings, if needed. Garnish with coriander and serve hot.

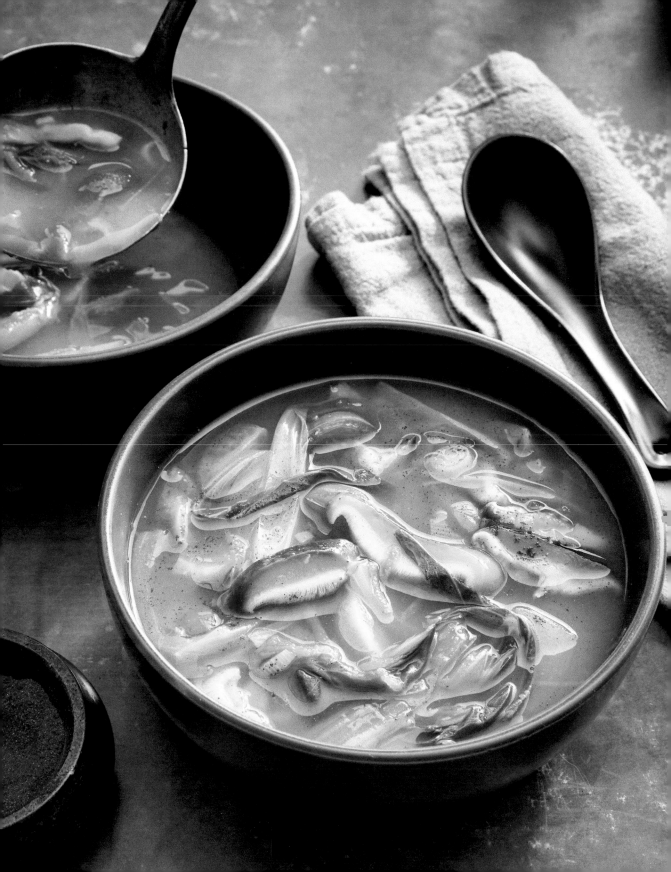

THREE-BEAN SOUP WITH TURMERIC AND LENTILS

MAKES: *4 to 6 servings*   DIFFICULTY: *Easy*

Turmeric casts a gorgeous golden glow on this hearty soup featuring lentils and three kinds of beans.

1 red onion, chopped

4 garlic cloves, thinly sliced

1 tablespoon ground turmeric

1 teaspoon ground coriander

½ teaspoon ground cumin

½ cup/100g dried brown lentils

7 cups/1.75 litres Light Vegetable Broth (page 214)

1½ cups/260g cooked* or 1 (400g) BPA-free tin or Tetra Pak salt-free red kidney beans, drained and rinsed

1½ cups/250g cooked* or 1 (400g) BPA-free tin or Tetra Pak salt-free chickpeas, drained and rinsed

1½ cups/260g cooked* or 1 (400g) BPA-free tin or Tetra Pak salt-free cannellini beans, drained and rinsed

6 cups/150g chopped spinach

1 cup/60g chopped fresh parsley

1 bunch spring onions, finely chopped

2 tablespoons chopped fresh mint, or 2 teaspoons dried

¼ teaspoon ground black pepper

Super-Charged Spice Blend (page 211)

Heat ¼ cup/60ml water in a large pot over a medium heat. Add the onion and garlic and cook for 5 minutes, to soften. Stir in the turmeric, coriander, cumin and lentils. Add the Light Vegetable Broth and bring to the boil.

Lower the heat to a simmer and add the kidney beans, chickpeas and cannellini beans. Cover and cook until the lentils are tender, 30 to 40 minutes. Add the spinach, parsley, spring onions, mint, black pepper and Super-Charged Spice Blend to taste and continue to cook for 10 minutes. Taste and adjust the seasonings, if needed. Serve hot.

Turn to the Legumes and Grains Cooking Charts *on pages 218–221 for instruction, if needed.*

BEANS AND PERIPHERAL VASCULAR DISEASE

Legumes – beans, chickpeas, split peas, and lentils – are an excellent source of vitamins, minerals, fibre and antioxidants.[23] In terms of nutrition density, they may give the biggest bang for the buck,[24] benefitting excess body weight, insulin resistance, high cholesterol, inflammation, and oxidative stress,[25] making them an important part of heart disease prevention.[26] Meet my Daily Dozen requirement of a minimum of three daily servings, and your heart will thank you.

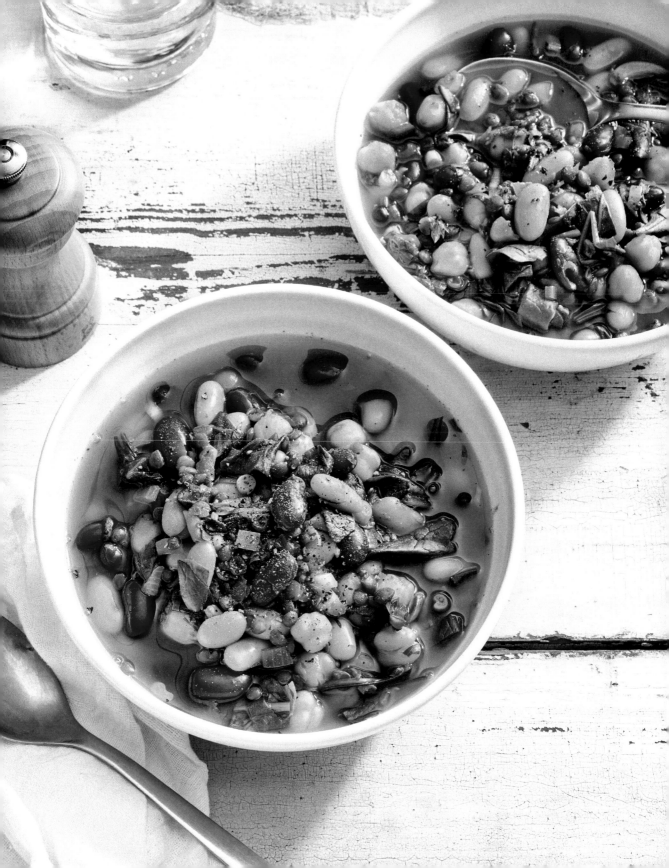

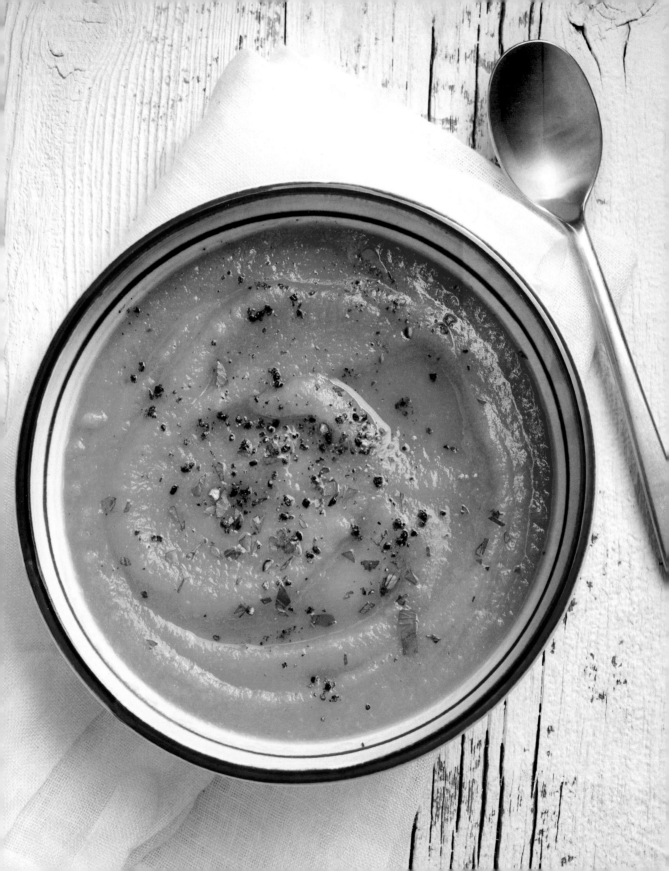

GINGER CARROT SOUP

MAKES: *4 servings*   DIFFICULTY: *Easy*

Fresh ginger perfectly complements the flavour of the carrots in this rich soup that can be enjoyed hot, warm or chilled. Feeling adventurous? To change up the flavour, add a teaspoon (or more) of your favourite curry powder or paste.

1 small onion, chopped

2 garlic cloves, chopped

1½ pounds/675g carrots, chopped

1 apple, cored and coarsely chopped

2 teaspoons grated fresh ginger, or to taste

¼ teaspoon ground black pepper

4 cups/1 litre Light Vegetable Broth (page 214)

1 tablespoon white miso paste

1 tablespoon apple cider vinegar

Optional garnishes: snipped fresh chives, chopped fresh parsley, or coarsely ground nigella seeds

Heat ¼ cup/60ml of water in a large pot over a medium heat. Add the onion and cook until softened, stirring occasionally, about 5 minutes. Add the garlic and carrots and cook for 5 minutes longer, stirring occasionally. Stir in the apple, ginger, black pepper and Light Vegetable Broth. Lower the heat to a simmer. Cover and cook until the carrots are soft, about 30 minutes.

Ladle ¼ cup/60ml of the hot broth into a small bowl or cup, add the miso paste, and stir until blended. Add the miso mixture to the soup along with the apple cider vinegar.

Working in batches, transfer the soup to a blender and blend until smooth. Taste and adjust the seasonings, if needed. Return the pureed soup to the pot and heat until hot, if needed. To serve, ladle the soup into bowls and top with your choice of optional garnishes.

CHEESY BROCCOLI SOUP

MAKES: *4 servings*   DIFFICULTY: *Easy*

We eat first with our eyes, and the lovely green broccoli florets against a backdrop of cheesy broth will have you wanting to eat with your mouth, too. If you prefer a smoother soup, you can puree all or part of the cooked broccoli, but I find it more satisfying to bite into broccoli florets with every spoonful of soup.

---

1 small onion, chopped

2 garlic cloves, finely chopped

1 celery stalk, chopped

6 cups/1.5 litres Light Vegetable Broth (page 214)

6 cups/425g small broccoli florets

1 cup/175g cooked* salt-free cannellini beans, drained and rinsed

¾ cup/115g raw cashews, soaked in boiling water for 30 minutes and then drained

1 (¼-inch/5mm) piece fresh turmeric, grated, or ¼ teaspoon ground

⅓ cup/45g nutritional yeast

1 tablespoon apple cider vinegar

1 teaspoon white miso paste

1 teaspoon smoked paprika

Ground black pepper

Heat ¼ cup/60ml of water in a large pot over a medium heat. Add the onion, garlic and celery and cook for 5 minutes. Add 2 cups/500ml of the Light Vegetable Broth and bring to the boil. Lower the heat to low and simmer until the vegetables are tender, about 5 minutes longer.

Transfer the soup mixture to a high-powered blender and blend until smooth. Transfer the pureed soup mixture back to the pot. Add the remaining 4 cups/1 litre of broth and bring to the boil. Add the broccoli and lower the heat to a simmer. Cook for 3 to 4 minutes, or until the broccoli is just softened. Do not overcook.

In the same blender (no need to clean it), combine 2 tablespoons of water and the cannellini beans, cashews, turmeric, nutritional yeast, apple cider vinegar, miso paste, paprika and black pepper to taste. Process until smooth. Taste and adjust the seasonings, if needed, until you reach your desired cheesy taste. Stir the bean mixture into the soup and heat over a low heat until hot.

Turn to the Legumes and Grains Cooking Charts *on pages 218–221 for instruction, if needed.*

ARE POLYAMIDE UTENSILS SAFE?

Polyamide plastics are often used to make kitchenware,[27] but polyamide chemicals can migrate into our food. Nearly one in three black plastic utensils tested exceeded the upper safety limit,[28] and up to about one in three were found to be contaminated with flame-retardant chemicals.[29] Opt for wooden and stainless-steel utensils instead.

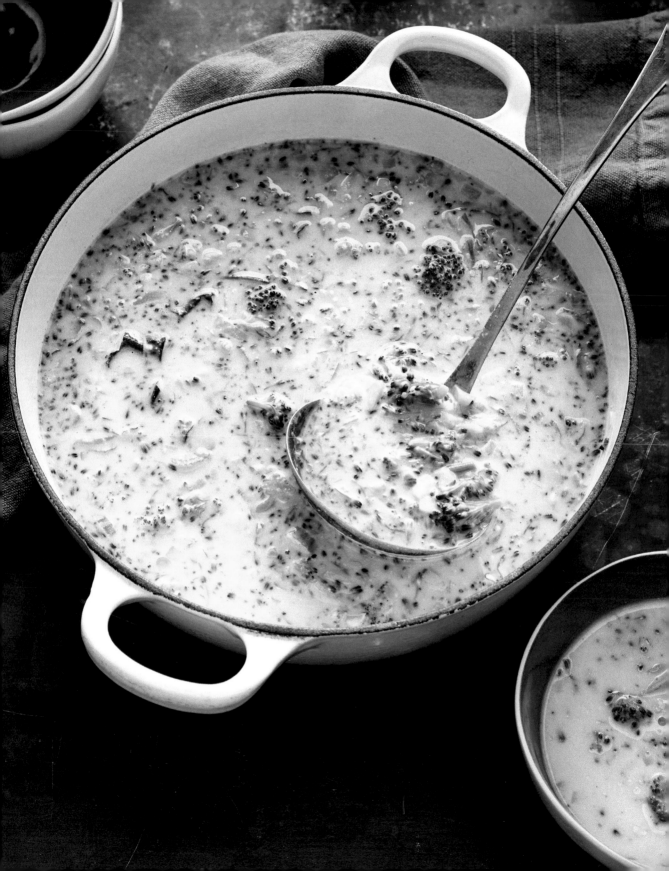

RATATOUILLE-INSPIRED PUY LENTIL SOUP

MAKES: *4 servings*   DIFFICULTY: *Moderate*

The famous French vegetable stew is the inspiration for this lentil soup, made with Puy lentils, of course. Herbes de Provence is a special blend of dried herbs that adds a unique depth of flavour and can be found in well-stocked supermarkets or online.

1 red onion, chopped

1 large orange or yellow pepper, de-seeded and cut into ½-inch/1cm dice

2 courgettes, cut into ½-inch/1cm dice

1 yellow squash, cut into ½-inch/1cm dice

3 to 4 garlic cloves, smashed

2 teaspoons Dr Greger's Special Spice Blend (page 212), or to taste

1 cup/200g Puy lentils

5 cups/1.25 litres Light Vegetable Broth (page 214)

2 pounds/900g ripe tomatoes, cored and halved

1 teaspoon herbes de Provence, or ½ teaspoon dried oregano and ½ teaspoon dried basil

¼ teaspoon ground black pepper or red pepper flakes

¼ cup/4 tablespoons chopped fresh basil

Preheat the oven to 220°C/425°F/gas mark 7. Line a large, rimmed baking tray with a silicone baking mat or baking parchment.

Spread the onion, pepper, courgette, yellow squash and garlic in a single layer on the prepared tray. (You may need two trays to fit all the vegetables.) Roast in the oven for 15 minutes. Remove from the oven and sprinkle with Dr Greger's Special Spice Blend. Use a metal spatula to flip the vegetables and return the tray(s) to the oven. Roast until the vegetables are tender and slightly caramelized, about 10 minutes longer. Remove from the oven and set aside.

While the vegetables are roasting, combine the lentils and Light Vegetable Broth in a large pot over a high heat. Bring to the boil, then lower the heat to a simmer, cover and cook until the lentils are just tender, about 20 minutes.

While the lentils are cooking, remove the roasted garlic from the baking tray and transfer to a food processor. Add the tomatoes and process until they are pureed and then add them to the pot. Stir in the herbes de Provence and black pepper.

Add the roasted vegetables to the pot and simmer over a low heat for 5 minutes to blend the flavours. Remove the pot from the heat. Stir in the fresh basil. Taste and adjust the seasonings, if needed. Serve hot.

Turn to the Legumes and Grains Cooking Charts *on pages 218–221 for instruction, if needed.*

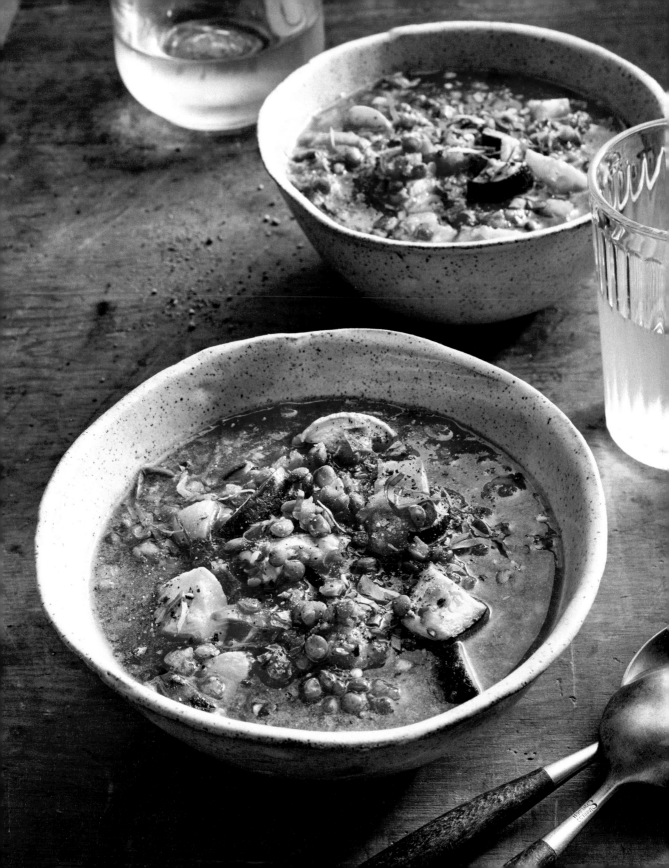

MY MINESTRONE

MAKES: *4 servings*   DIFFICULTY: *Easy*

Minestrone is a popular vegetable soup from Italy that is enjoyed around the world. My version is loaded with even more vegetables than usual and topped with a spoonful of Basil Pesto for added flavour.

1 large red onion, chopped

2 carrots, cut into thin rounds

3 garlic cloves, finely chopped

1 red pepper, de-seeded and chopped

1 courgette, cut into ¼-inch/5mm dice

1 (400g) BPA-free tin or Tetra Pak salt-free chopped tomatoes, undrained

2 tablespoons salt-free tomato puree

8 ounces/225g green beans, trimmed and cut into 2-inch/5cm pieces

1 teaspoon finely chopped fresh oregano, or ½ teaspoon dried

6 cups/1.5 litres Light Vegetable Broth (page 214)

½ teaspoon ground black pepper

3 cups/75g baby kale

1½ cups/250g cooked* or 1 (400g) BPA-free tin or Tetra Pak salt-free chickpeas, drained and rinsed

2 tablespoons Basil Pesto (page 215)

Heat ¼ cup/60ml of water in a large pot over a medium heat. Add the onion, carrots and garlic and cook for 5 minutes to soften. Add the pepper, courgette, tomatoes with their juices, tomato puree, green beans, oregano, Light Vegetable Broth and black pepper. Bring to the boil, then lower the heat to a simmer. Cover and cook until the vegetables are tender, about 20 minutes. Stir in the baby kale and chickpeas and cook for 10 minutes longer. Ladle the hot soup into bowls and top each with a spoonful of Basil Pesto. Serve hot.

＊*Turn to the* Legumes and Grains Cooking Charts *on pages 218–221 for instruction, if needed.*

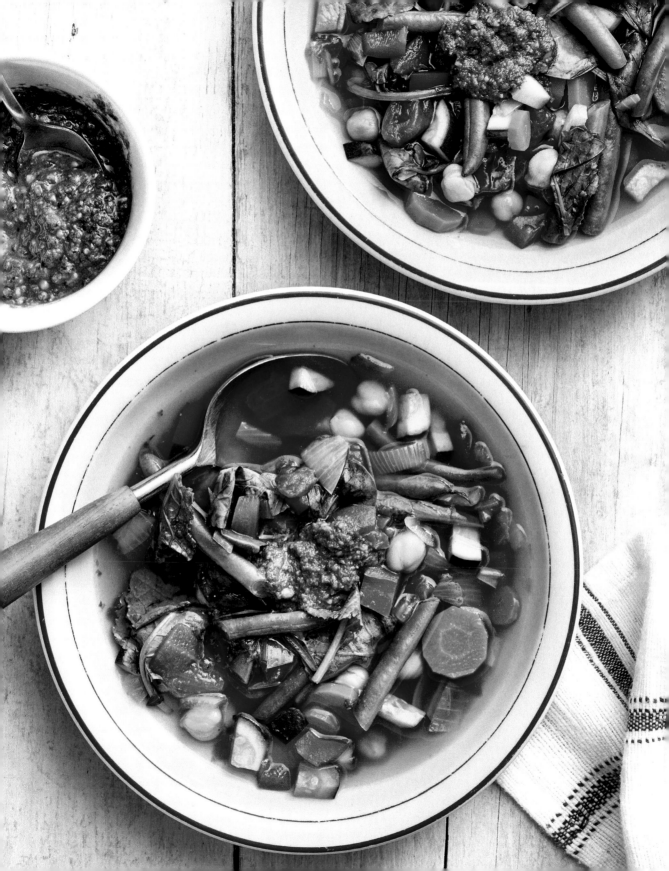

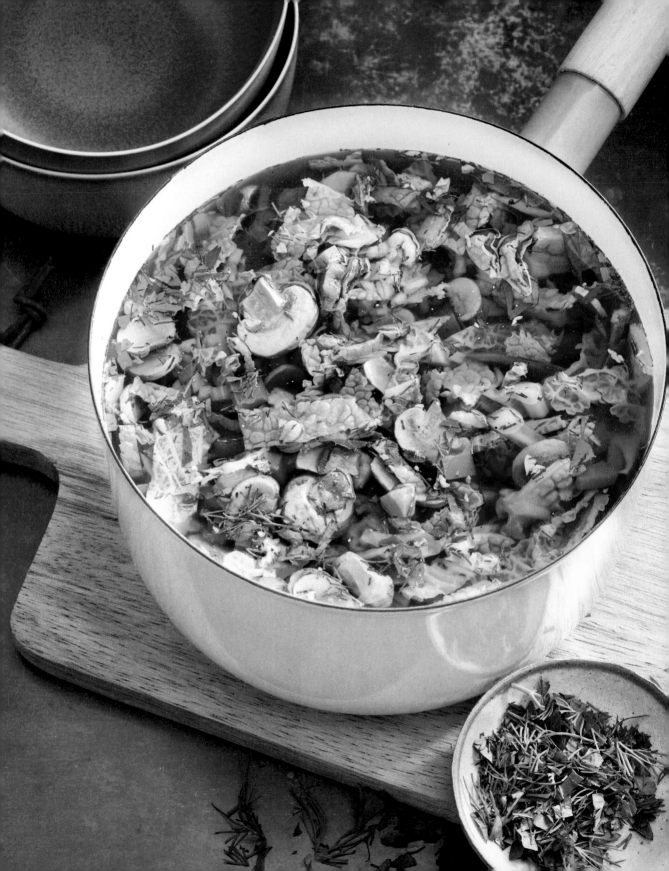

MUSHROOM BARLEY SOUP

MAKES: *4 to 6 servings*   DIFFICULTY: *Easy*

Be sure to use pot barley (groats) instead of pearl barley to get the most nutrients.

1 small red onion, chopped

1 carrot, chopped

1 celery stalk, chopped

¾ cup/150g pot barley (groats), washed, rinsed, and drained

8 cups/2 litres Light Vegetable Broth (page 214)

3 cups/300g chopped savoy cabbage

1 pound/450g baby portobello or white button mushrooms, sliced or diced

2 teaspoons Dr Greger's Special Spice Blend (page 212), or to taste

1½ teaspoons dried thyme

Ground black pepper

Chopped fresh parsley or dill

Heat ¼ cup/60ml of water in a large pot over a medium heat. Add the onion, carrot and celery. Cover and cook until softened, about 5 minutes, stirring occasionally. Add the barley and Light Vegetable Broth. Bring to the boil, then lower the heat to a simmer, cover and cook for 30 minutes. Stir in the cabbage, mushrooms, Dr Greger's Special Spice Blend, thyme and black pepper to taste. Cover and simmer until the barley and vegetables are tender, about 30 minutes longer. Taste and adjust the seasonings, if needed. To serve, ladle the soup into bowls and garnish with parsley or dill.

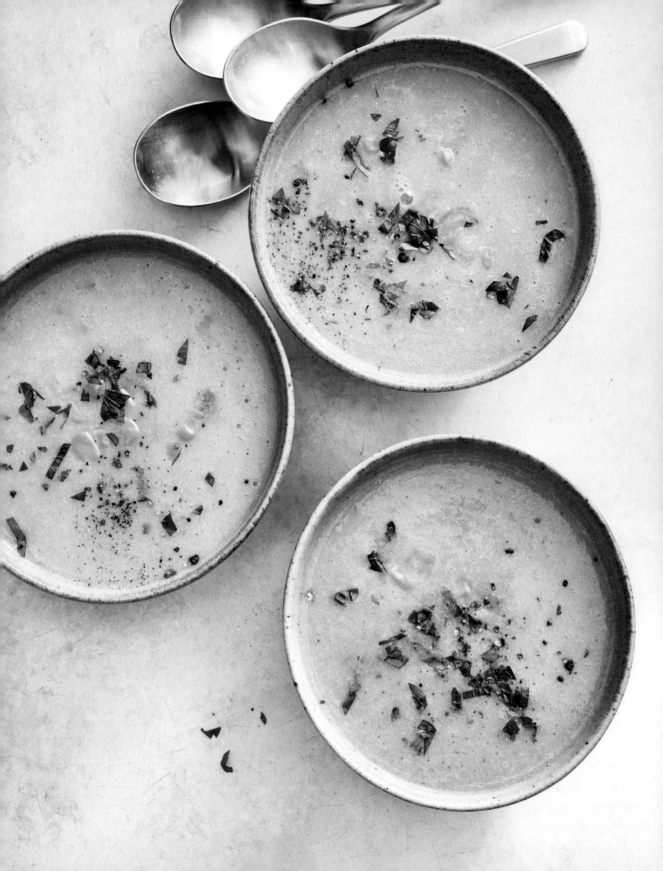

CORN CHOWDER

MAKES: *4 servings*   DIFFICULTY: *Easy*

This chowder can be as thick and creamy as you like, depending on how much of the soup you puree. Don't forget to put the Salt-Free Hot Sauce on the table for those who want to add a little heat.

1 onion, chopped

2 celery stalks, chopped

2 floury potatoes, diced

¼ cup/35g nutritional yeast

½ teaspoon smoked paprika

½ teaspoon dried thyme

¼ teaspoon ground black pepper

4 cups/1 litre Light Vegetable Broth (page 214)

1 pound/450g fresh or thawed frozen sweetcorn

2 teaspoons white miso paste

2 teaspoons fresh lemon juice

1 tablespoon finely chopped fresh parsley

Salt-Free Hot Sauce (page 216) (optional)

Heat ¼ cup/60ml of water in a large pot over a medium heat. Add the onion, celery and potatoes. Cover and cook, stirring occasionally, for 5 minutes, or until softened. Stir in the nutritional yeast, paprika, thyme, black pepper and Light Vegetable Broth. Bring to the boil, then lower the heat to low, stir in the sweetcorn and simmer for 20 minutes, or until the vegetables are tender.

Scoop 2 cups/500ml of the soup solids into a high-powered blender, add the miso paste, and blend until smooth. Stir the pureed mixture back into the soup. Add the lemon juice, then taste and adjust the seasonings, if needed. If you prefer a thicker chowder, puree another cup/250ml of soup solids and add it back to the pot. Heat the soup until hot and serve sprinkled with parsley and with Salt-Free Hot Sauce on the side (if using).

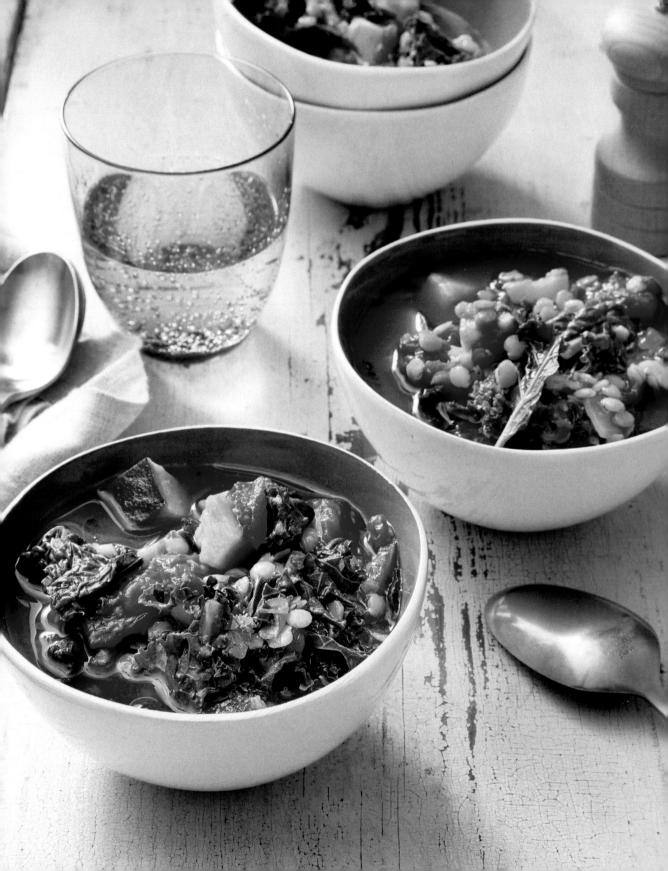

CURRIED LENTIL AND KALE SOUP

MAKES: *4 servings*   DIFFICULTY: *Easy*

This simple soup is so full of flavour, it tastes as if it took hours to make. Spinach, chard or other dark leafy greens may be substituted for the kale if desired.

1 red onion, chopped

2 cups/270g diced sweet potato or de-seeded butternut squash

1 garlic clove, finely chopped

1 tablespoon grated fresh ginger

1 tablespoon curry powder

1 teaspoon ground coriander

½ teaspoon ground cumin

¼ teaspoon ground black pepper

1 cup/200g dried red lentils, picked over and rinsed

5 cups/1.25 litres Light Vegetable Broth (page 214)

1 (400g) BPA-free tin or Tetra Pak salt-free finely chopped tomatoes

3 cups/200g chopped kale

1 teaspoon fresh lemon juice

Super-Charged Spice Blend (page 211)

1 teaspoon coarsely ground nigella seeds

Heat ¼ cup/60ml of water in a large pot over a medium heat. Add the onion, sweet potato and garlic. Cover and cook until softened, about 8 minutes. Stir in the ginger, curry powder, coriander, cumin and black pepper. Add the lentils and Light Vegetable Broth and bring to the boil. Lower the heat to low and simmer until the lentils and vegetables are tender, stirring occasionally, about 30 minutes. Stir in the tomatoes and kale and continue to cook until the kale is tender, 10 to 15 minutes. Stir in the lemon juice and Super-Charged Spice Blend to taste. Adjust the seasonings, if needed. Serve hot, sprinkled with nigella seeds.

TUSCAN WHITE BEAN SOUP WITH ROASTED FENNEL

MAKES: *4 servings*   DIFFICULTY: *Moderate*

The slightly anise flavour of fennel is a welcome addition to this soup. Pureeing half of the beans and leaving the rest whole adds creaminess to the broth while still keeping some texture for a more complex soup.

1 large fennel bulb

1 small onion, chopped

4 garlic cloves, finely chopped

3 cups/525g cooked* or 2 (400g) BPA-free tins or Tetra Paks salt-free cannellini beans, drained and rinsed

4 cups/1 litre Light Vegetable Broth (page 214)

2 teaspoons chopped fresh rosemary, plus more to serve (optional)

½ teaspoon ground fennel seeds

¼ teaspoon ground black pepper

1 teaspoon fresh lemon juice

Preheat the oven to 220°C/425°F/gas mark 7. Line a rimmed baking tray with a silicone mat or baking parchment.

Cut off the bottom and top of the fennel bulb, reserving some fronds for garnish, if you wish. Slice the bulb in half, lengthways; then cut lengthways into ¼-inch/5mm slices. Spread out the fennel pieces on the prepared baking tray. Roast in the oven for about 30 minutes, or until tender and browned, turning once about halfway through.

Heat ¼ cup/60ml of water in a large pot over a medium heat. Add the onion and garlic. Cover and cook, stirring occasionally, until the onion is tender, about 8 minutes. Add half of the cannellini beans, Light Vegetable Broth, rosemary, ground fennel seeds and black pepper and bring to the boil. Lower the heat to a simmer and cook for 10 minutes. Remove from the heat and allow the soup to cool slightly.

Use a hand blender to puree the soup or, working in batches, transfer the soup to a blender and puree before returning the soup to the pot. Stir in the remaining half of the beans and return to a simmer to heat through for about 10 minutes, stirring occasionally. Stir in the lemon juice; then taste and adjust the seasonings, if needed.

To serve, ladle the soup into bowls and top with a portion of the roasted fennel and more chopped fresh rosemary or reserved chopped fennel fronds, if desired.

*Turn to the Legumes and Grains Cooking Charts on pages 218–221 for instruction, if needed.

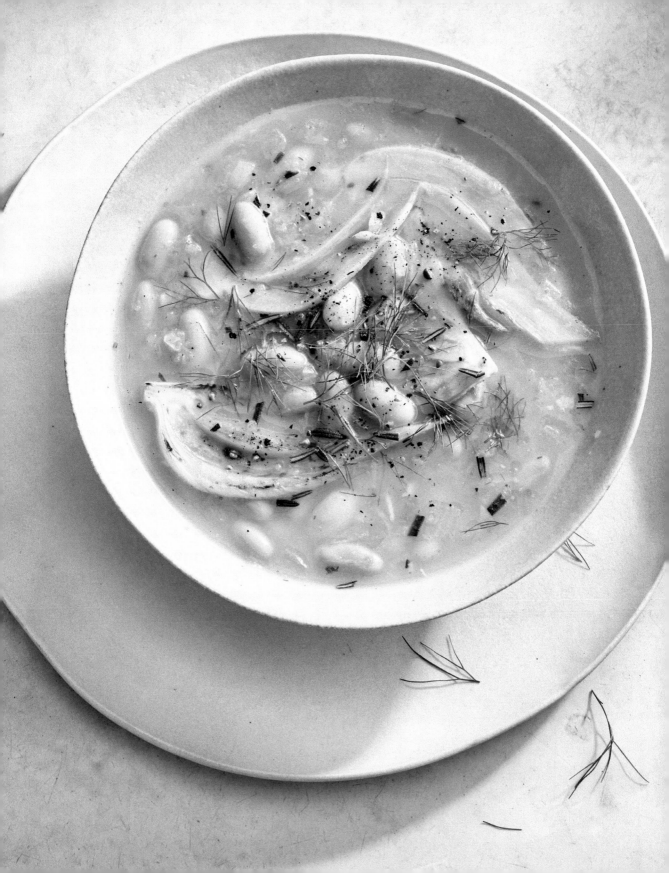

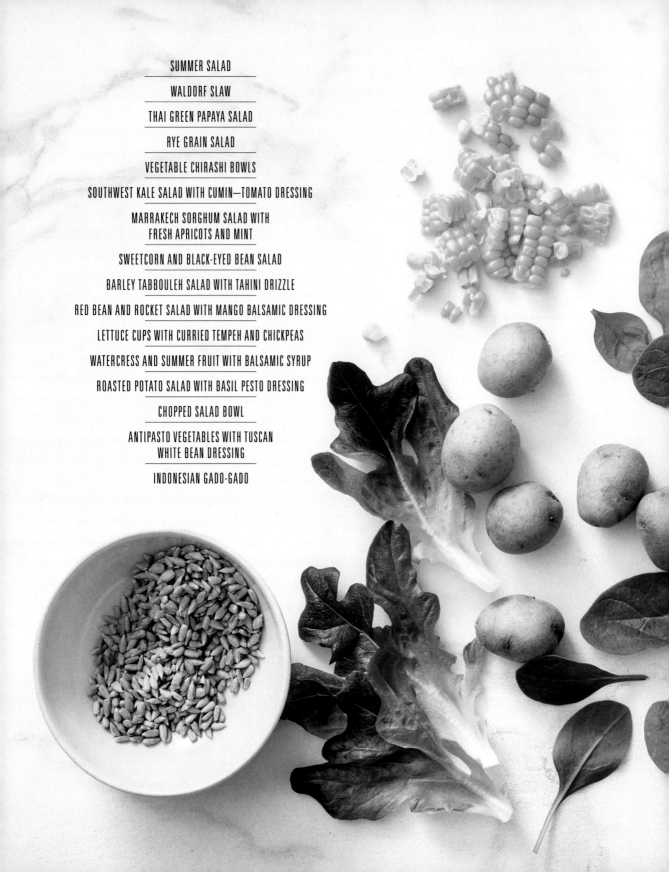

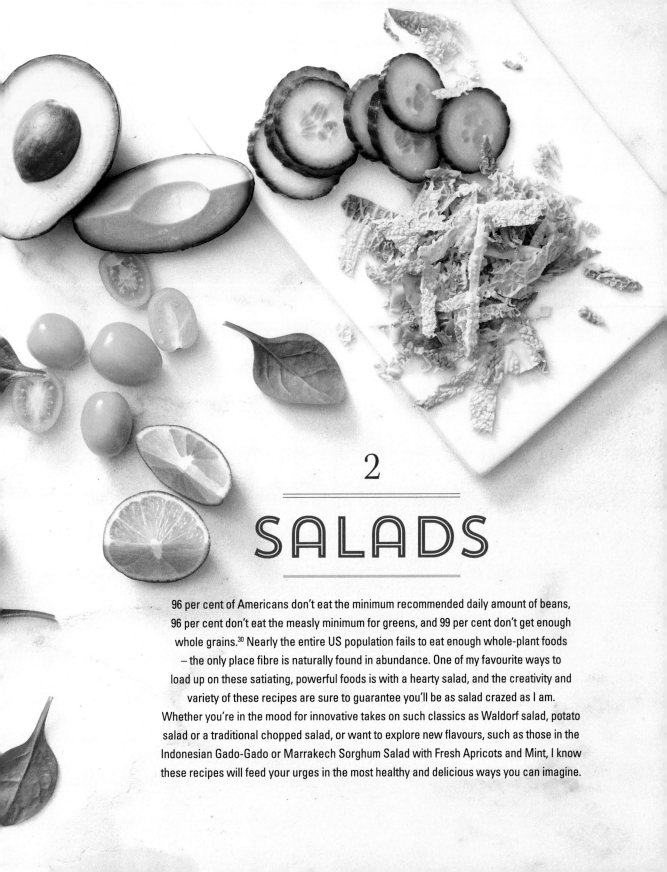

2

SALADS

96 per cent of Americans don't eat the minimum recommended daily amount of beans, 96 per cent don't eat the measly minimum for greens, and 99 per cent don't get enough whole grains.[30] Nearly the entire US population fails to eat enough whole-plant foods – the only place fibre is naturally found in abundance. One of my favourite ways to load up on these satiating, powerful foods is with a hearty salad, and the creativity and variety of these recipes are sure to guarantee you'll be as salad crazed as I am. Whether you're in the mood for innovative takes on such classics as Waldorf salad, potato salad or a traditional chopped salad, or want to explore new flavours, such as those in the Indonesian Gado-Gado or Marrakech Sorghum Salad with Fresh Apricots and Mint, I know these recipes will feed your urges in the most healthy and delicious ways you can imagine.

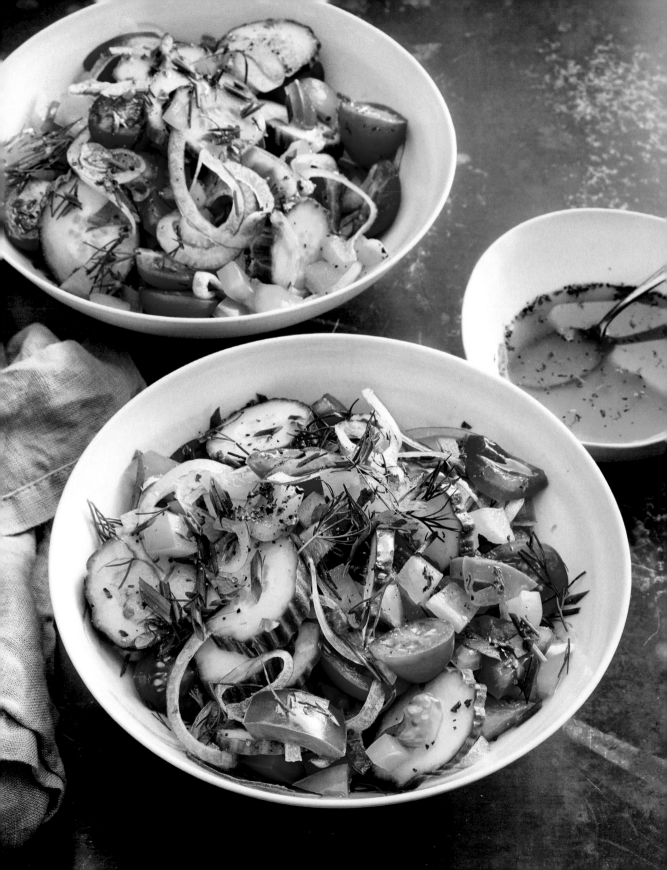

SUMMER SALAD

MAKES: *4 servings*   **DIFFICULTY:** *Easy*

This refreshing salad is delicious year-round, but I especially love it when summer produce is at its peak.

3 ripe tomatoes, cut into ½-inch/1cm dice, or 3 cups/450g cherry tomatoes, halved

1 cucumber, ends trimmed and cut into ¼-inch/5mm slices

1 small yellow pepper, de-seeded and cut into ½-inch/1cm dice

¼ cup/30g thinly sliced red onion

3 tablespoons chopped fresh herbs, such as parsley, dill, basil or chives

⅓ cup/75ml apple cider vinegar

1 teaspoon white miso paste

¼ teaspoon dried basil

¼ teaspoon dried oregano

¼ teaspoon ground black pepper

In a large bowl, combine the tomatoes, cucumber, pepper, onion and fresh herbs. Set aside.

In a small bowl, whisk together ⅓ cup/75ml of water with the apple cider vinegar, miso paste, dried basil, dried oregano and black pepper. Pour the dressing over the vegetables and toss gently to coat. Serve.

WALDORF SLAW

MAKES: *4 servings*   DIFFICULTY: *Easy*

The classic Waldorf salad reimagined as a tasty slaw. You'll still find the apples, walnuts, celery and grapes, but in this version, hold the heavy mayo and enjoy more veggies.

3 to 4 Gala or Fuji apples, cored and cut into ½-inch/1cm dice

2 tablespoons fresh lemon juice

2 tablespoons apple cider vinegar

1 soft pitted date, soaked for 10 minutes in hot water and then drained (optional)

1 teaspoon grated fresh ginger

1 teaspoon white miso paste

¼ teaspoon ground black pepper

3 cups/300g shredded cabbage

1 large carrot, grated

½ cup/50g seedless red grapes, halved

1 celery stalk, finely chopped

½ cup/60g chopped walnuts

2 spring onions, finely chopped

Place the diced apples in a large bowl and toss lightly with the lemon juice to coat.

Scoop out ½ cup/50g of the diced apple mixture and transfer to a blender. Add 2 tablespoons of water, the apple cider vinegar, date (if using), ginger, miso paste, and black pepper and blend until smooth. Set the dressing aside.

To the large bowl of diced apple, add the cabbage, carrot, grapes, celery, walnuts and spring onions. Add the dressing to the slaw and toss gently to combine. Taste and adjust the seasonings, if needed.

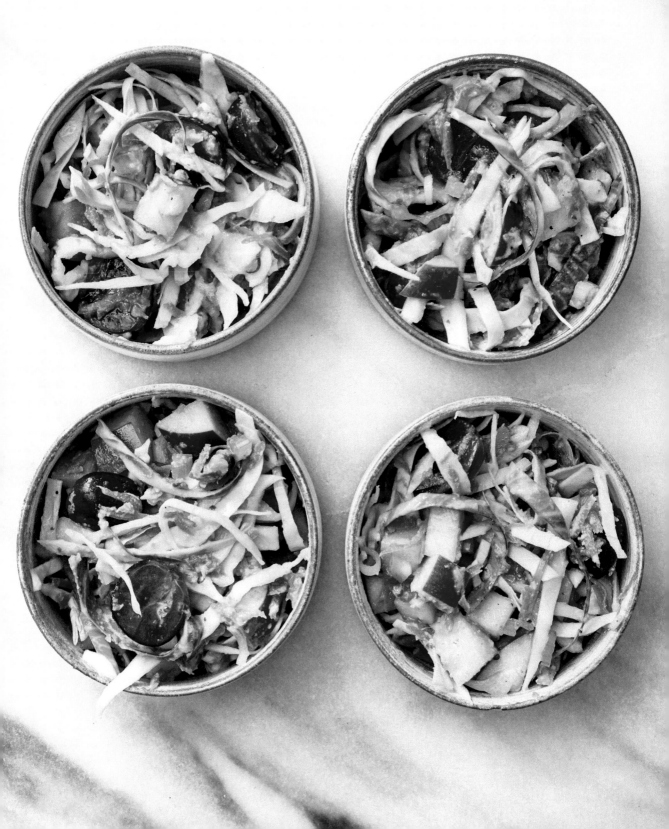

THAI GREEN PAPAYA SALAD

MAKES: *4 servings*   DIFFICULTY: *Easy*

No need to go out to a Thai restaurant to enjoy this flavour-packed salad. With this simple (and simply delicious) recipe, you can make it at home. Grate the papaya and carrot on a mandoline slicer or box grater. If you can't get hold of green papaya, you could try cucumber and/or shredded cabbage. Leave off the red pepper flakes if you don't want the heat, or add even more if you really like to spice things up.

Zest and juice of 1 lime

2 garlic cloves, finely chopped

2 tablespoons apple cider vinegar

2 teaspoons grated fresh ginger

1 teaspoon white miso paste

1 teaspoon Date Syrup (page 217)

¼ teaspoon red pepper flakes, or to taste

1 large green papaya, peeled, de-seeded and grated

1 carrot, peeled and grated

1½ cups/165g green beans, cut into 1½-inch/4cm pieces and lightly steamed

1 cup/150g cherry tomatoes, halved lengthways

2 spring onions, finely chopped

⅓ cup/40g crushed unsalted roasted peanuts

In a small bowl, combine 2 tablespoons of water, the lime zest and juice, garlic, apple cider vinegar, ginger, miso paste, Date Syrup and red pepper flakes. Set the dressing aside.

In a large bowl, combine the papaya, carrot, green beans, tomatoes and spring onions. Pour the dressing on the salad and toss to combine. Sprinkle with the peanuts and serve.

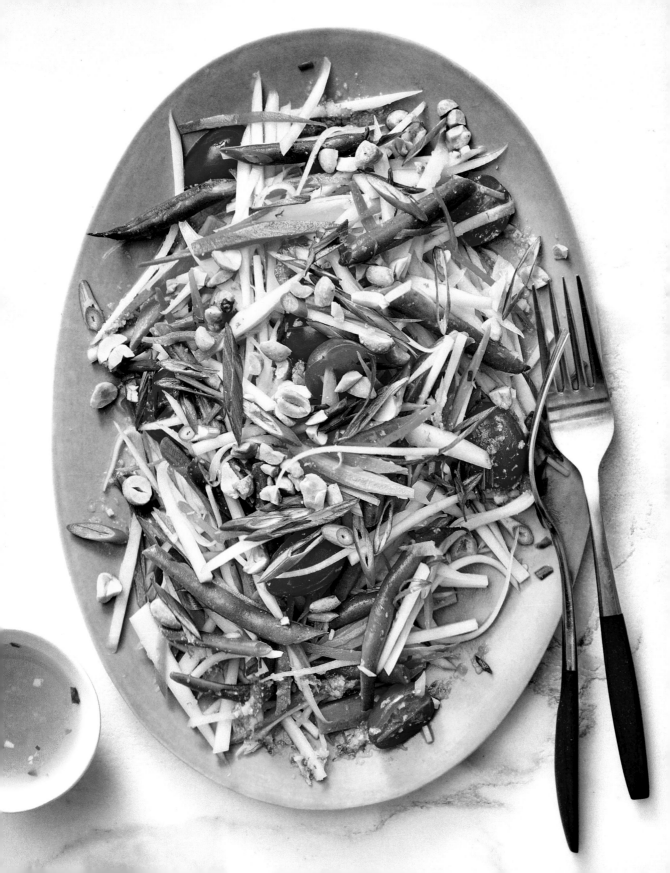

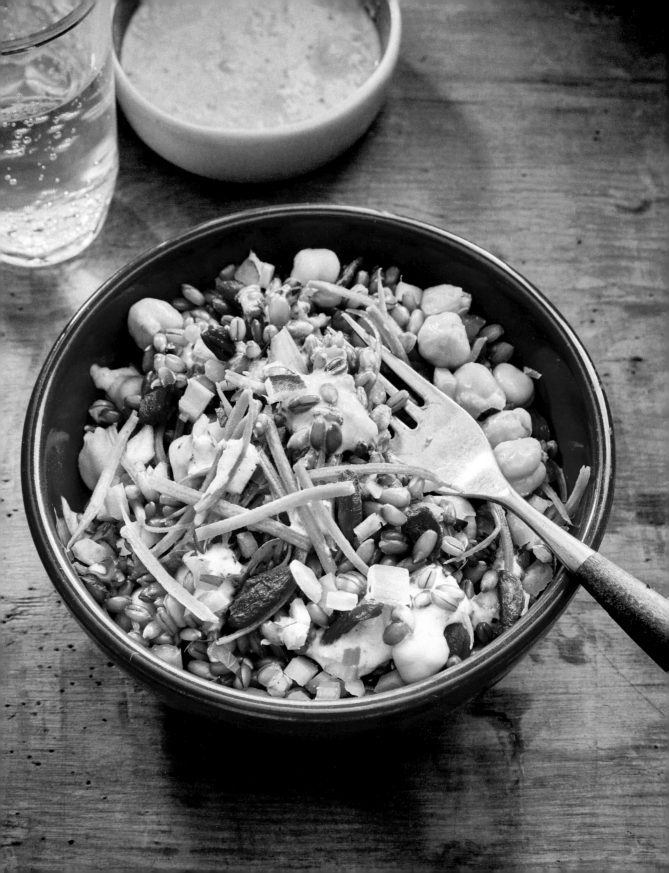

RYE GRAIN SALAD

MAKES: *4 servings*   DIFFICULTY: *Moderate*

Hearty, chewy rye grains are featured in this salad made with chickpeas, veggies and a zesty mustard dressing. They may take a moment to cook, but rye grains are well worth the time. Your palate and your health will thank you.

1 cup/170g rye grains, soaked overnight in water and then drained

2 large carrots, grated

½ small red onion, finely chopped

1½ cups/150g finely chopped celery

1½ cups/250g cooked* or 1 (400g) BPA-free tin or Tetra Pak salt-free chickpeas, drained and rinsed

3 tablespoons dried goji berries

½ cup/50g sliced almonds

¼ cup/15g chopped fresh coriander or parsley

¼ teaspoon ground black pepper

1 orange, peeled and quartered

2 teaspoons fresh lemon juice

2 tablespoons balsamic or sherry vinegar

1 tablespoon white miso paste

1 soft pitted date, soaked for 10 minutes in hot water and then drained

1 garlic clove, finely chopped

2 teaspoons salt-free wholegrain mustard

Cook* the rye grains in a pressure cooker or a pot on the stovetop. Set aside to cool.

Transfer the cooled rye grains to a large bowl. Add the carrots, onion, celery, chickpeas, goji berries, almonds, coriander and black pepper. Set aside.

In a blender, combine the orange, lemon juice, vinegar, miso paste, date, garlic and mustard. Blend until smooth. Taste and adjust the seasonings, if needed.

Pour the dressing over the rye mixture and toss gently to coat. Cover and set aside for 30 minutes to allow the flavours to blend. If not serving right away, store, covered, in the refrigerator.

Turn to the Legumes and Grains Cooking Charts *on pages 218–221 for instruction, if needed.*

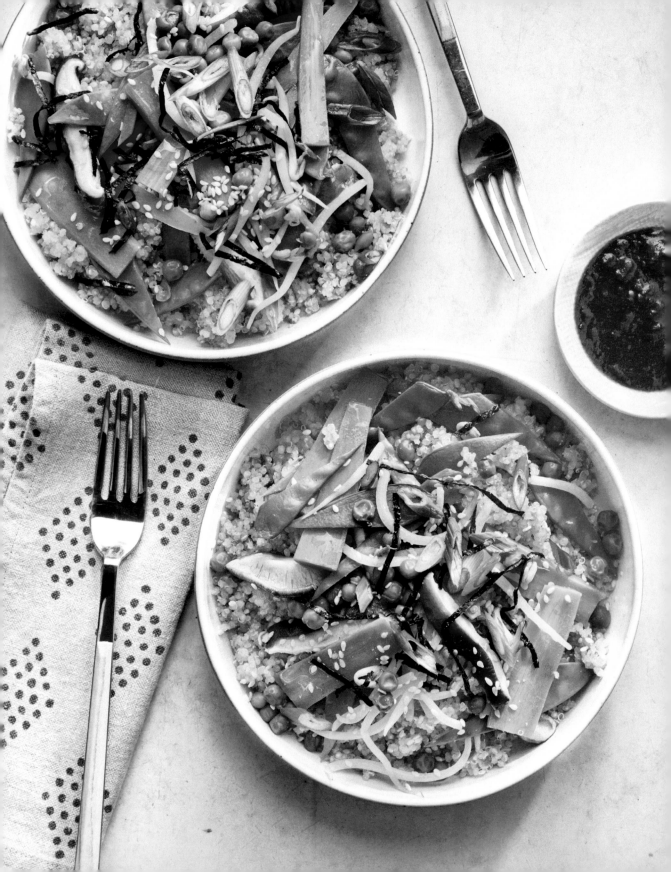

VEGETABLE CHIRASHI BOWLS

MAKES: *4 servings*   DIFFICULTY: *Moderate*

The refreshing Japanese 'scattered sushi' salad known as *chirashi-zushi* typically calls for raw fish on a bed of rice. This lighter version features vegetables instead of fish, and quinoa replaces the sticky rice. The salad is topped with nori strips as a nod to the sea.

1 cup/170g uncooked quinoa, well rinsed

2 tablespoons rice vinegar

1 tablespoon white miso paste

1 carrot, cut into thin, 2-inch/5cm strips

1 cup/75g de-stemmed and thinly sliced shiitake mushrooms

1 cup/150g frozen peas

1 cup/100g trimmed and diagonally cut 1-inch/2.5cm pieces of mange tout

1 cup/100g fresh bean sprouts

1 spring onion, finely chopped

1 tablespoon sesame seeds

1 sheet nori, cut into 2-inch x ¼-inch/5cm x 5mm strips

Umami Sauce Redux (page 212)

Bring 2 cups/500ml of water to the boil in a saucepan. Add the quinoa and lower the heat to low. Cover and simmer until the water is absorbed, about 15 minutes. Drain well to remove any excess moisture and set aside for 5 minutes to make sure all the water is absorbed. Sprinkle the cooked quinoa with the vinegar and toss gently to combine. Transfer the quinoa to a shallow serving bowl and set aside to cool to room temperature.

In a saucepan over a medium heat, combine 1 cup/250ml of water with the miso paste, stirring to dissolve the miso. Bring the water to a simmer, add the carrot, mushrooms and peas and cook until softened, about 2 minutes. Add the mange tout and bean sprouts and cook until the mange tout turn bright green, about 1 minute longer. Remove from the heat. Drain well and rinse under cold water to stop the cooking process and cool the vegetables.

Spread ('scatter') the vegetables over the quinoa. Sprinkle with the spring onion, sesame seeds and nori strips. Serve at room temperature with the Umami Sauce Redux on the table to add as desired.

THE BEST WAY TO COOK VEGETABLES

Healthy antioxidant plant pigments appear to be sensitive to really high temperatures, so avoid frying, especially deep-frying.[31] Blanching – submerging veggies into boiling water for three minutes, then running them under cold water – was even better than boiling; and steam blanching – steaming veggies for three minutes, then letting them cool off – may be even better.[32]

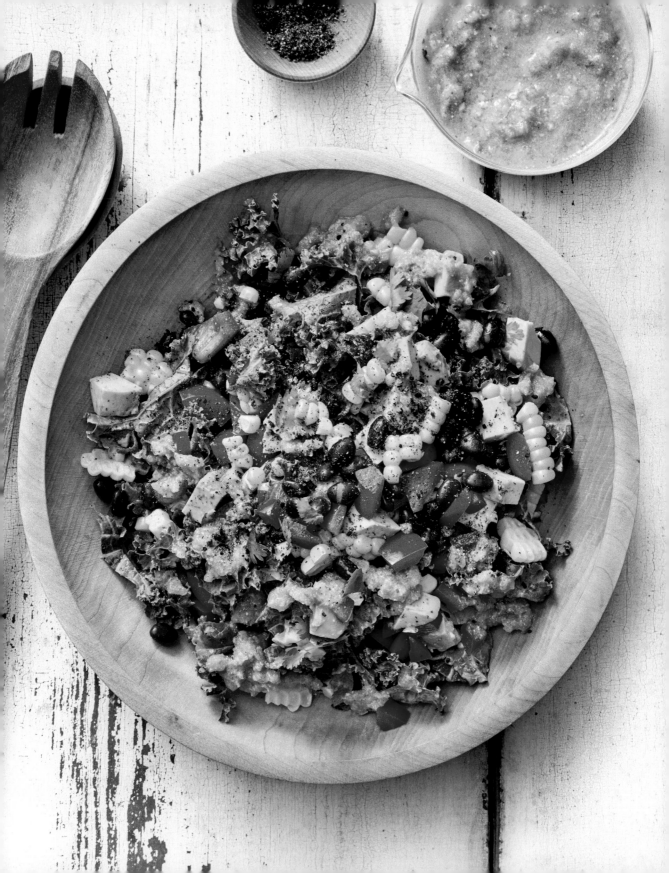

SOUTHWEST KALE SALAD WITH CUMIN-TOMATO DRESSING

MAKES: *4 servings*   DIFFICULTY: *Easy*

Favourite flavours of the Southwest combine in this hearty main-dish salad starring kale and black beans.

DRESSING

1 large ripe tomato, cored and quartered

1 garlic clove, crushed

¼ cup/60ml apple cider vinegar

2 tablespoons nutritional yeast

1 teaspoon ground cumin

½ teaspoon dried oregano

½ teaspoon white miso paste

½ teaspoon Super-Charged Spice Blend (page 211), or to taste

¼ teaspoon ground black pepper

SALAD

1 large bunch kale, tough stems removed

1½ cups/250g cooked* or 1 (400g) BPA-free tin or Tetra Pak salt-free black beans, drained and rinsed

1 small red pepper, de-seeded and diced

1½ cups/260g fresh or thawed frozen sweetcorn

1 ripe Hass avocado, peeled, pitted, and diced

¼ cup/4 tablespoons chopped fresh coriander or parsley

TO SERVE

Coarsely ground nigella seeds

FOR THE DRESSING: In a blender, combine all the dressing ingredients. Blend well until smooth, scraping down the sides as needed. Add up to ¼ cup/60ml of water if the dressing is too thick, or add more tomato if too thin. Taste to adjust the seasonings.

FOR THE SALAD: Finely chop the kale and place in a large bowl. Add the black beans, pepper, corn, avocado and coriander.

TO SERVE: Pour on as much of the dressing on the salad as desired and toss gently to combine. Sprinkle the top with nigella seeds.

✶Turn to the Legumes and Grains Cooking Charts on pages 218–221 for instruction, if needed.

EFFECTS OF AVOCADOS ON INFLAMMATION

Researchers compared ice cream to the same calories of avocado. Unlike the ice cream, the avocado, despite being packed with calories and fat, did not produce a rise in oxidative or inflammatory activity. Sugar is okay in fruit form because it comes naturally pre-packaged with phytonutrients. Similarly, the fat in whole plant foods, such as nuts and avocados, comes pre-packaged with 'a rich matrix of phytochemicals and therefore does not demonstrate the same potential for oxidative damage.'[33]

MARRAKECH SORGHUM SALAD WITH FRESH APRICOTS AND MINT

MAKES: *4 servings*   DIFFICULTY: *Moderate*

Sorghum has its origins in Africa, so it's only fitting to use it in a vibrant Moroccan salad seasoned with Ras el Hanout and fresh mint leaves. Dried apricots would be more typical in a salad like this, but fresh apricots really add something special.

SORGHUM

1½ cups/300g sorghum, soaked overnight in water

1 carrot, grated

½ cup/30g chopped fresh parsley

2 tablespoons finely chopped chives or spring onions

1 tablespoon sherry vinegar

1 teaspoon Ras el Hanout (recipe opposite)

DRESSING

1 teaspoon Ras el Hanout

2 garlic cloves, crushed

2 tablespoons almond butter

1 tablespoon fresh lemon juice

1 teaspoon white miso paste

SALAD

½ cup/50g sliced almonds or sunflower seeds

4 fresh ripe apricots, pitted and cut into wedges

1 cup/50g chopped fresh mint leaves

TO SERVE

Chopped romaine lettuce and rocket

FOR THE SORGHUM: Drain and rinse the soaked sorghum. Cook* the sorghum in a pot on the stovetop or a pressure cooker. Transfer the cooked sorghum to a large bowl and set aside to cool. Add the remaining ingredients for the sorghum. Toss gently to combine.

FOR THE DRESSING: In a blender, combine ¼ cup/60ml of water with all the dressing ingredients. Blend until smooth.

FOR THE SALAD: Add the dressing to the bowl of seasoned sorghum. Add the almonds, apricots and mint leaves and toss gently to coat.

TO SERVE: Serve immediately on a bed of chopped lettuce and rocket. If not serving right away, store in an airtight container without the apricots and mint leaves. Add those final ingredients just before serving.

Turn to the Legumes and Grains Cooking Charts *on pages 218–221 for instruction, if needed.*

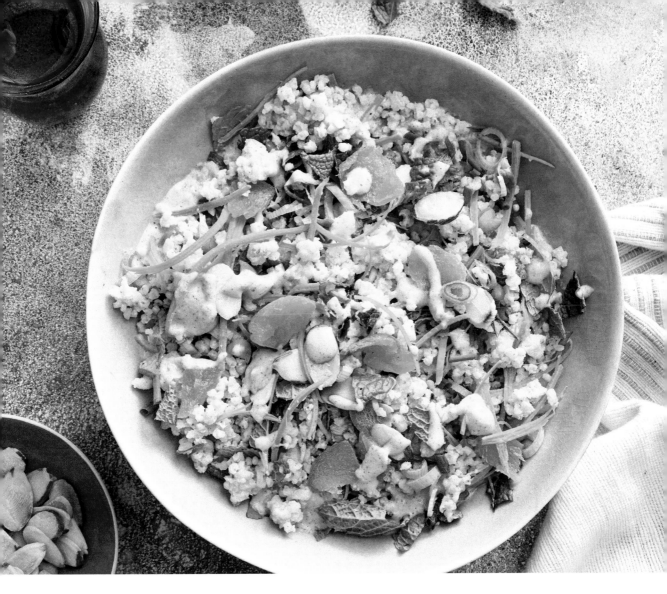

1½ teaspoons ground ginger

1½ teaspoons ground coriander seeds

1 teaspoon ground turmeric

1 teaspoon ground cinnamon

1 teaspoon ground cumin

½ teaspoon ground allspice

½ teaspoon ground cardamom

½ teaspoon ground anise or
fennel seeds

½ teaspoon ground black pepper

¼ teaspoon cayenne

¼ teaspoon ground cloves

RAS EL HANOUT

MAKES: *3 tablespoons*   DIFFICULTY: *Easy*

Meaning 'head of the shop', this Moroccan spice blend is
available in spice shops and online, or you can make your own.

Place all the ingredients in a small bowl and stir to combine well. Store
in an airtight container at room temperature.

SWEETCORN AND BLACK-EYED BEAN SALAD

MAKES: *4 servings*   DIFFICULTY: *Easy*

A variety of textures, colours and flavours makes this salad a hit at potlucks and picnics. Enjoy it as a side or as a main-dish salad.

SALAD

3 cups/500g cooked* or 2 (400g) BPA-free tins or Tetra Paks salt-free black-eyed beans, drained and rinsed

2 cups/350g fresh or thawed frozen sweetcorn

¼ cup/40g finely chopped red onion

1 small red pepper, de-seeded and diced

1 ripe Hass avocado, peeled, pitted and diced

1 small jalapeño pepper, de-seeded and finely chopped (optional)

⅓ cup/20g chopped fresh coriander

DRESSING

1 large ripe tomato, cored and quartered

¼ cup/60ml fresh lemon juice

½ teaspoon smoked paprika

½ teaspoon chilli powder

1 teaspoon Super-Charged Spice Blend (page 211), or to taste

Ground black pepper

TO SERVE

1 tablespoon sunflower seeds

FOR THE SALAD: In a large bowl, combine the black-eyed beans, sweetcorn, onion, pepper, avocado, jalapeño (if using) and coriander.

FOR THE DRESSING: In a small blender, combine the tomato, lemon juice, paprika, chilli powder, Super-Charged Spice Blend and black pepper.

TO SERVE: Pour the dressing over the salad and toss gently to coat. Sprinkle the sunflower seeds on top and serve.

Turn to the Legumes and Grains Cooking Charts on pages 218–221 for instruction, if needed.

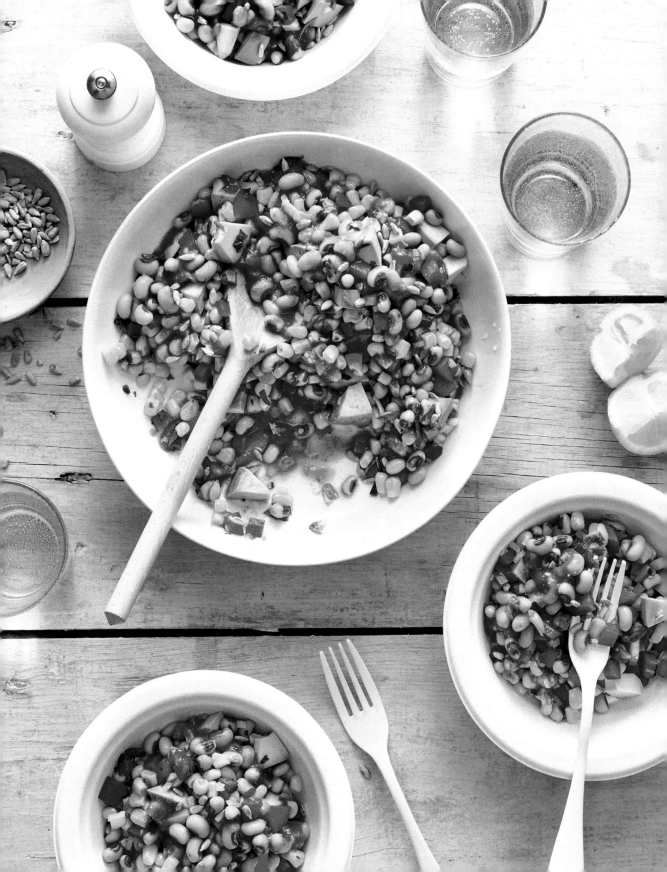

BARLEY TABBOULEH SALAD
WITH TAHINI DRIZZLE

MAKES: *4 servings*   DIFFICULTY: *Moderate*

Intact barley stands in for cracked bulgur in this hearty salad, but you can use another whole grain if you prefer. This recipe is a great way to make use of any leftover cooked whole grains you may have on hand. A drizzle of tahini sauce adds a unique depth of flavour to the salad.

TABBOULEH

¾ cup/150g pot barley, soaked overnight in water and then drained

2 ripe plum tomatoes, chopped

1 cucumber, peeled, de-seeded and chopped

1½ cups/330g cooked* or 1 (400g) BPA-free tin or Tetra Pak salt-free chickpeas, drained and rinsed

2 bunches parsley, finely chopped

½ cup/25g chopped fresh mint

2 spring onions, finely chopped

4 tablespoons fresh lemon juice

1 teaspoon white miso paste

½ teaspoon garlic powder

¼ teaspoon ground cumin

Super-Charged Spice Blend (page 211)

TAHINI SAUCE

1 garlic clove, crushed

3 tablespoons tahini

1 tablespoon fresh lemon juice

1 teaspoon white miso paste

Pinch of ground cumin

TO SERVE

6 cups/200g mesclun greens

Coarsely ground nigella seeds

FOR THE TABBOULEH: Cook* the barley in a pressure cooker or a pot on the stovetop. Drain off any excess water and set aside to cool.

Place the cooked barley in a large bowl. Add the tomatoes, cucumber, chickpeas, parsley, mint and spring onions. Set aside.

In a small bowl, combine the lemon juice, miso paste, garlic powder, cumin and Super-Charged Spice Blend to taste. Mix well.

Pour the dressing over the barley mixture and mix gently to combine. Cover and set aside for 20 minutes to allow the flavours to blend. If not serving right away, refrigerate until needed.

FOR THE TAHINI SAUCE: In a small blender, combine all the tahini sauce ingredients plus ¼ cup/60ml of water and blend until smooth. For a thinner sauce, add a little more water, 1 tablespoon at a time.

TO SERVE: Spoon the tabbouleh onto plates or into shallow bowls lined with mesclun greens. Drizzle with the tahini sauce and sprinkle with the nigella seeds.

✻Turn to the Legumes and Grains Cooking Charts *on pages 218–221 for instruction, if needed.*

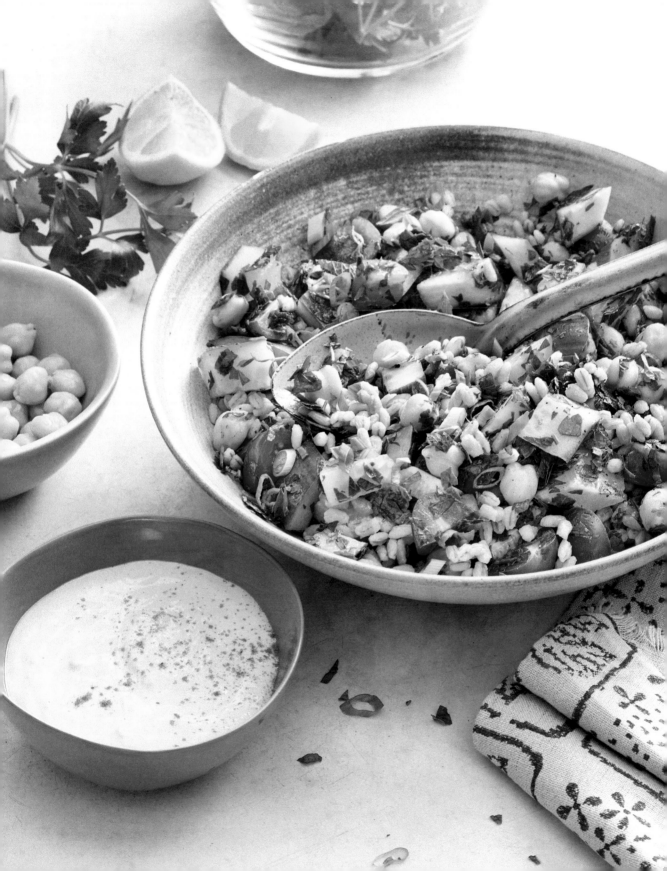

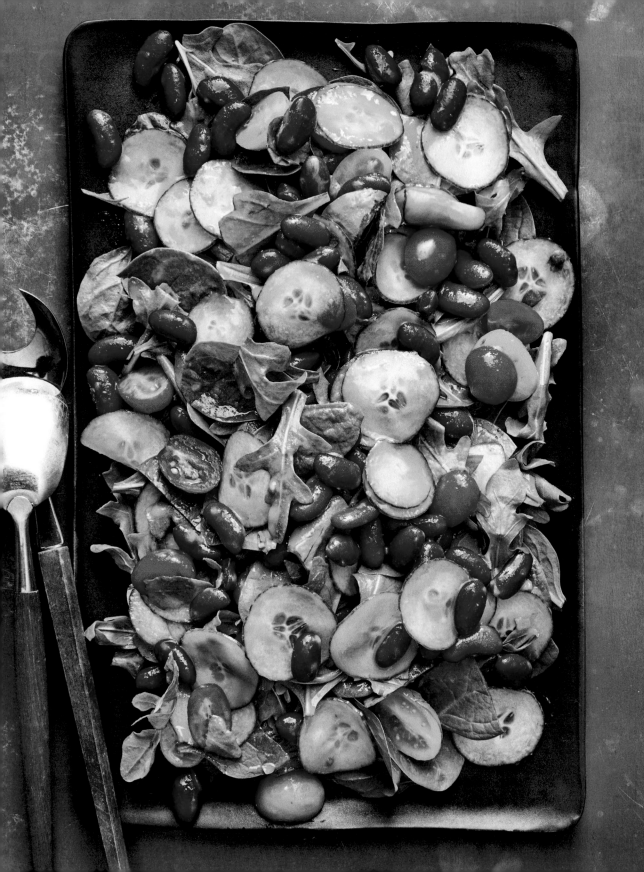

RED BEAN AND ROCKET SALAD WITH MANGO BALSAMIC DRESSING

MAKES: *4 servings*   DIFFICULTY: *Easy*

If you like to mix up your greens a bit, swap out some of the rocket for 2 cups/100g of chopped watercress or red leaf lettuce, or add them to the salad for even more glorious greens.

1 ripe mango, peeled, pitted, and coarsely chopped

2 tablespoons balsamic vinegar

1 tablespoon finely chopped spring onion

2 teaspoons finely chopped fresh parsley or coriander

1 teaspoon white miso paste

1 (¼-inch/5mm) piece fresh turmeric, grated, or ¼ teaspoon ground

6 cups/150g chopped rocket or baby spinach leaves

1½ cups/260g cooked* or 1 (400g) BPA-free tin or Tetra Pak salt-free red kidney beans or adzuki beans, drained and rinsed

1 cucumber, thinly sliced

1 cup/150g cherry tomatoes, halved lengthways

In a blender, combine the mango, vinegar, spring onion, parsley, miso paste and turmeric. Blend until smooth. Set aside.

In a large bowl, combine the rocket, beans, cucumber and tomatoes. Pour the dressing over the salad and toss gently to combine. Serve immediately.

*Turn to the Legumes and Grains Cooking Charts *on pages 218–221 for instruction, if needed.*

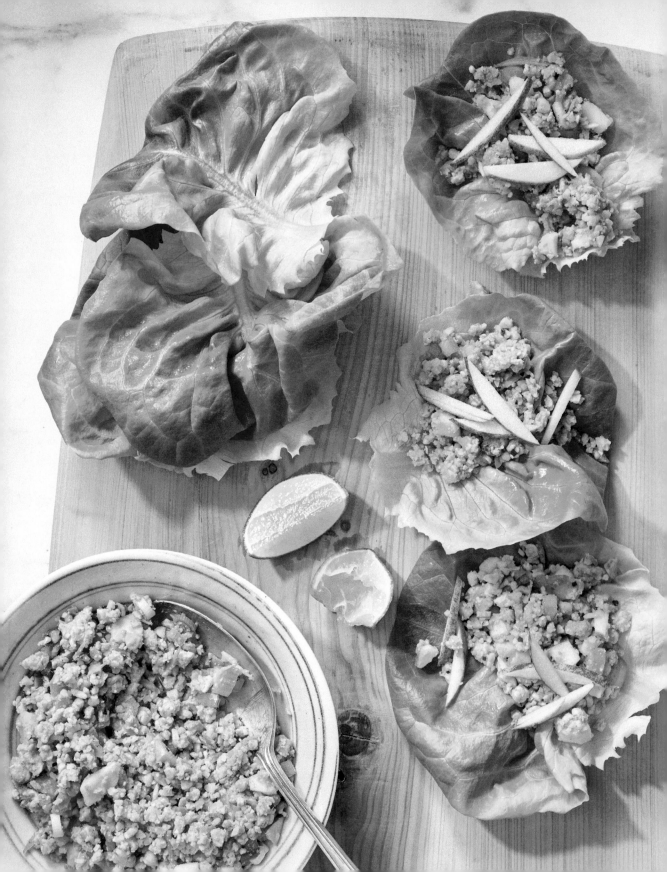

LETTUCE CUPS WITH CURRIED TEMPEH AND CHICKPEAS

MAKES: *4 servings*   DIFFICULTY: *Easy*

Two tips for you: If you make the curried tempeh and chickpeas in advance of when you want to serve this dish, the flavours will have time to merge and get even bolder. And small, soft lettuce leaves make the best cups for holding the salad.

8 ounces/225g tempeh, steamed for 20 minutes, then cooled and crumbled

1½ cups/250g cooked* or 1 (400g) BPA-free tin or Tetra Pak salt-free chickpeas, drained and rinsed

½ cup/50g chopped celery

⅓ cup/60g grated carrot

1 Fuji or Gala apple, cored and coarsely chopped

1 tablespoon chopped spring onion

1½ teaspoons curry powder, or to taste

2 teaspoons fresh lemon juice

1 teaspoon white miso paste

8 to 10 whole leaves round lettuce

In a food processor or a large bowl, combine the crumbled tempeh, chickpeas (lightly mashed if using a bowl instead of a food processor), celery, carrot, apple, spring onion, curry powder, lemon juice and miso paste. Add 3 tablespoons of water. Pulse or mix until combined. If using a food processor, pulse less if you want the salad to be chunky or pulse more if you prefer a smoother salad mixture. If using a bowl, the mixture will be very chunky. Taste and adjust the seasonings, if needed.

To assemble, spoon the curried tempeh and chickpeas into the lettuce leaf cups and serve immediately.

Turn to the Legumes and Grains Cooking Charts *on pages 218–221 for instruction, if needed.*

SHOULD WOMEN WITH FIBROIDS AVOID SOYA?

About one in four women will suffer from fibroids, most commonly with excessively heavy periods and pain or pressure.[34] Is there a link to soya? No. The amount of soya phytoestrogen in three to five cups of soya milk a day had no significant effect on the frequency or growth of fibroids.[35]

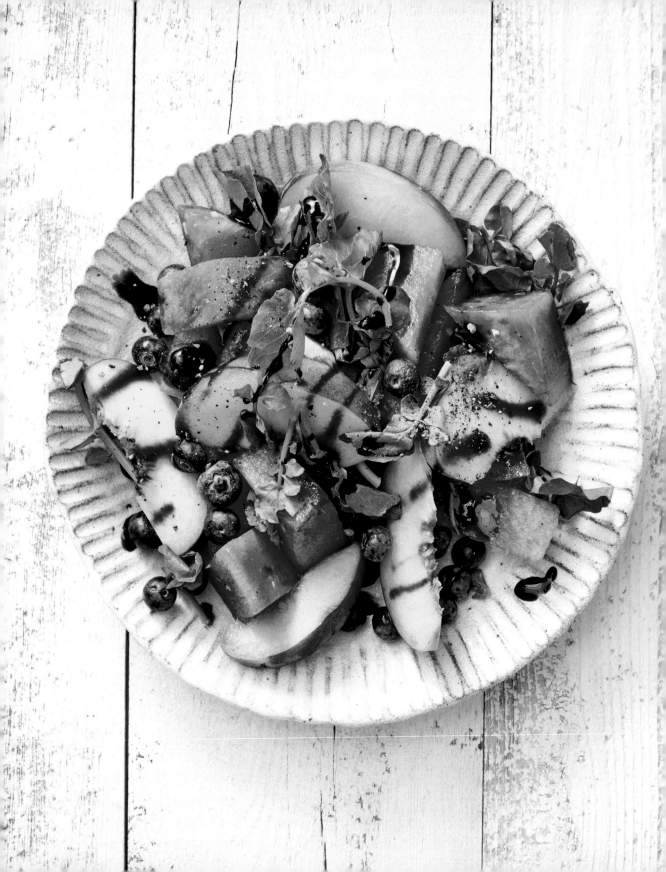

WATERCRESS AND SUMMER FRUIT WITH BALSAMIC SYRUP

MAKES: *4 servings*   DIFFICULTY: *Easy*

Balsamic syrup brings out the sweetness of the fruit. Make this refreshing salad when summer fruit and watercress are at their peak.

3 cups/450g (1-inch/2.5cm) diced or balled (with a melon baller) watermelon

3 ripe peaches, pitted and cut into thin wedges or diced

1 cup/100g fresh blueberries

2 teaspoons fresh lemon juice

2 bunches watercress, tough stems removed, coarsely chopped

Balsamic Syrup (page 215)

Coarsely ground black pepper

In a large bowl, combine the watermelon, peaches, blueberries and lemon juice. Toss to combine. Add the watercress and toss again.

To serve, drizzle the salad with as much Balsamic Syrup as desired and sprinkle with coarsely ground black pepper to taste.

BENEFITS OF BLUEBERRIES FOR ARTERY FUNCTION

Eating blueberries provides chronic benefits in terms of reduced artery stiffness and a boost in natural killer cells, one of our natural defences against viral infections and cancer.[36]

And, when we eat blueberries, we're not only improving our artery function, but we're also feeding our good bacteria. Win-win![37]

ROASTED POTATO SALAD WITH BASIL PESTO DRESSING

MAKES: *4 servings*   DIFFICULTY: *Easy*

Roasting the potatoes for this salad adds amazing flavour and texture, and the Basil Pesto dressing sends it over the top.

1½ pounds/675g waxy or new potatoes, cut into 1-inch chunks

2 tablespoons white wine vinegar

¼ teaspoon onion powder

¼ teaspoon garlic powder

¼ teaspoon ground black pepper

2 celery stalks, finely chopped

1 carrot, grated

1 cup/175g cooked* or BPA-free tinned or Tetra Pak salt-free cannellini beans, drained and rinsed

3 spring onions, finely chopped

1 tablespoon fresh lemon juice

1 tablespoon white balsamic vinegar

1 cup/250ml Basil Pesto (page 215), or to taste

Preheat the oven to 220°C/425°F/gas mark 7. Line a rimmed baking tray with a silicone mat or baking parchment.

In a bowl, combine the potatoes with the vinegar, onion powder, garlic powder and black pepper, tossing gently to coat. Spread the potatoes on the prepared tray. Roast in the oven until tender and lightly browned, about 25 minutes, turning once about halfway through.

Transfer the roasted potatoes to a large serving bowl and allow to cool. Once the potatoes are cool, add the celery, carrot, beans, spring onions, lemon juice, vinegar and the Basil Pesto and toss gently to combine.

Turn to the Legumes and Grains Cooking Charts *on pages 218–221 for instruction, if needed.*

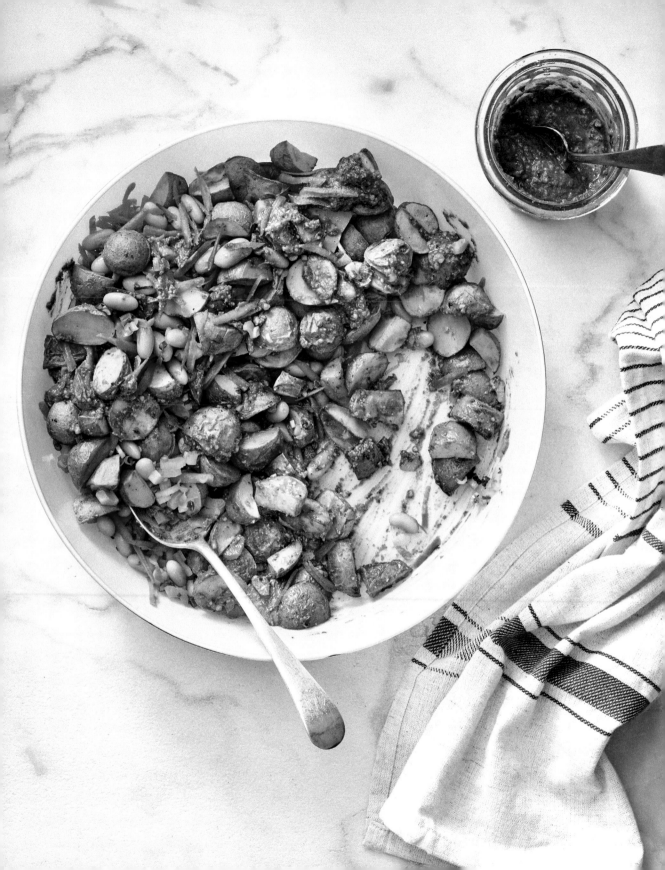

CHOPPED SALAD BOWL

MAKES: *4 servings*   DIFFICULTY: *Easy*

This chopped salad is loaded with fresh vegetables. Get creative with the recipe and incorporate what you have on hand, or add what you've always wanted to try. The possibilities are endless.

DRESSING

2 tablespoons tahini

2 tablespoons apple cider vinegar

1 tablespoon fresh lemon juice

1 tablespoon nutritional yeast

1 teaspoon white miso paste

1 teaspoon dried basil or another herb of your choice, such as thyme, marjoram or tarragon

¼ teaspoon onion powder

¼ teaspoon garlic powder

¼ teaspoon ground black pepper

¼ teaspoon ground cumin (optional)

SALAD

1 head romaine lettuce, chopped into bite-size pieces

1 cucumber, peeled, halved lengthways and chopped

2 cups/350g steamed small broccoli or cauliflower florets

1 sweet potato, roasted and cooled, then diced

1 large ripe tomato, chopped

1 yellow pepper, de-seeded and chopped

1 Hass avocado, peeled, pitted and diced

3 radishes, chopped

1 tablespoon sunflower seeds or hemp hearts

FOR THE DRESSING: Combine all the dressing ingredients plus 3 tablespoons of water in a small blender or food processor and blend until smooth.

FOR THE SALAD: In a large bowl, combine all the salad ingredients, except the sunflower seeds. Shake or stir the dressing to recombine, and then add it to the salad, tossing gently. Sprinkle with sunflower seeds and serve.

ARE PRE-CUT VEGETABLES JUST AS HEALTHY?

Endotoxins come from bacteria, such as *E. coli*.[38] Most spoilage organisms cannot penetrate the surface barrier of plants to spoil the inner tissues, but once you cut them open, bacteria can gain access and vegetables can start to spoil in a matter of days.[39] What does this mean for pre-cut veggies? While it's better to eat pre-cut vegetables than no vegetables at all, slicing and dicing whole veggies yourself might be healthiest.

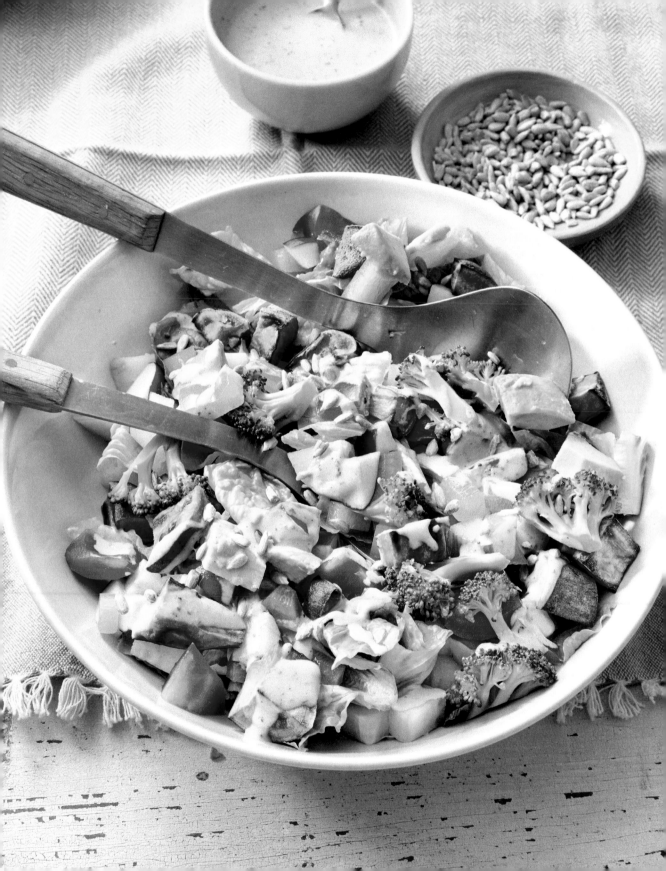

ANTIPASTO VEGETABLES WITH TUSCAN WHITE BEAN DRESSING

MAKES: *4 servings*   DIFFICULTY: *Easy*

This hearty dish is served at room temperature, so I like to roast the vegetables and make the dressing ahead of when I plan to enjoy it so I can just assemble its components right before serving.

VEGETABLES

1 red onion, cut into ½-inch/1cm slices

1 courgette, trimmed and cut lengthways into ¼-inch/5mm strips

1 yellow summer squash, trimmed and cut lengthways into ¼-inch/5mm strips

1 red pepper, de-seeded and cut into 1-inch/2.5cm strips

2 large portobello mushroom caps, gills scraped out and discarded, quartered or thickly sliced

2 cups/300g cherry tomatoes, halved

DRESSING

2 garlic cloves, coarsely chopped

2 tablespoons nutritional yeast

½ cup/90g cooked* or BPA-free tinned or Tetra Pak salt-free cannellini beans, drained and rinsed

1 (¼-inch/5mm) piece fresh turmeric, grated, or ¼ teaspoon ground

2 tablespoons white balsamic vinegar

1 tablespoon fresh lemon juice

2 teaspoons white miso paste

½ teaspoon salt-free mustard

1 tablespoon finely chopped fresh parsley

¾ teaspoon chopped fresh rosemary

½ teaspoon chopped fresh sage

Dr Greger's Special Spice Blend (page 212)

TO SERVE

3 cups/75g rocket

½ cup/15g fresh basil leaves, torn

FOR THE VEGETABLES: Preheat the oven to 220°C/425°F/gas mark 7. Line one or two large, rimmed roasting tins with silicone mats or baking parchment.

In separate groups, evenly place all the vegetables, except the tomatoes, in the prepared tin(s). Scatter the tomatoes over the piles of vegetables. Roast in the oven, turning once, until the vegetables are tender and nicely browned, about 10 minutes per side. Remove from the oven and allow to cool to room temperature.

FOR THE DRESSING: In a blender, combine all the dressing ingredients, adding Dr Greger's Special Spice Blend to taste, and blend until smooth. Taste and adjust the seasoning, if needed.

TO SERVE: Spread the rocket on a large platter. Arrange the cooled roasted vegetables in separate piles on top of the rocket and drizzle with the dressing. Sprinkle the fresh basil on top and serve.

✴Turn to the Legumes and Grains Cooking Charts *on pages 218–221 for instruction, if needed.*

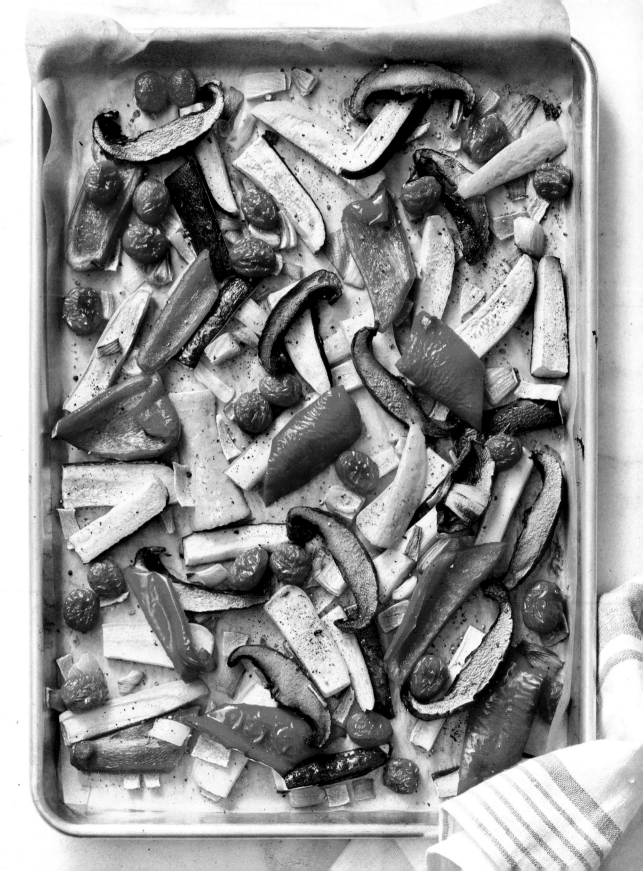

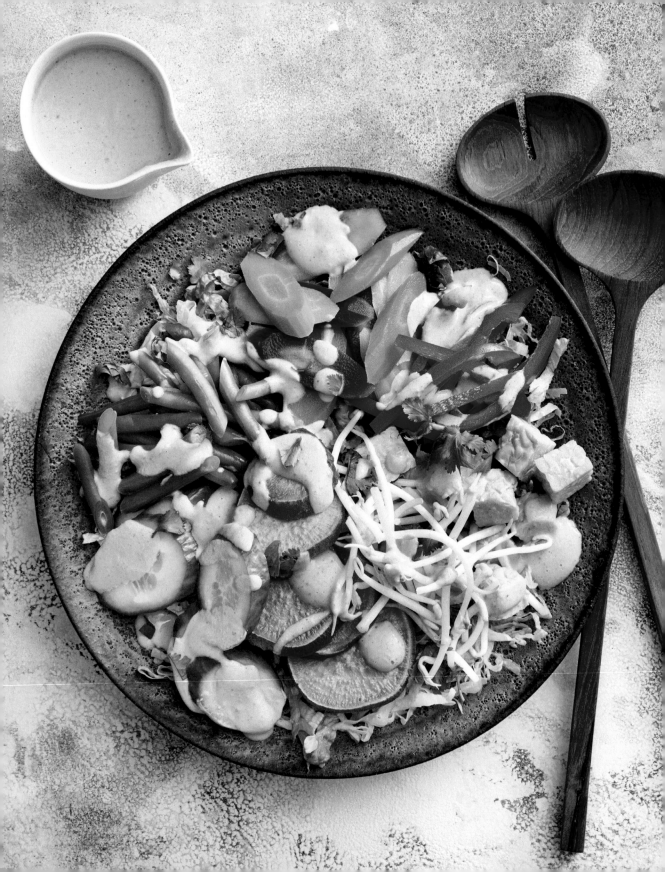

INDONESIAN GADO-GADO

MAKES: *4 servings*   DIFFICULTY: *Easy*

This popular Indonesian vegetable salad takes a little time to prepare all the components, but it's easy to assemble. Use more or less cayenne (or none at all) according to your own taste.

PEANUT SAUCE

1 garlic clove, crushed

1½ tablespoons grated fresh ginger

¼ to ½ teaspoon cayenne, to taste

1 teaspoon ground coriander

½ teaspoon garlic powder

½ teaspoon onion powder

1 tablespoon lemon juice

2 tablespoons apple cider vinegar

⅓ cup/60g smooth unsalted peanut butter

2 tablespoons Umami Sauce Redux (page 212)

1 cup/250ml hot water, or as needed

SALAD

1 large sweet potato, cut into ¼-inch/5mm slices

8 ounces/225g green beans, trimmed and cut into 1½-inch/4cm pieces

2 carrots, thinly sliced

TO SERVE

Shredded lettuce or spinach

1 cucumber, cut into ½-inch/1cm slices

1 red pepper, de-seeded and thinly sliced

¾ cup/75g bean sprouts

8 ounces/225g steamed tempeh, cut into ½-inch/1cm dice

Chopped fresh coriander

2 to 3 tablespoons roasted unsalted peanuts

FOR THE PEANUT SAUCE: Combine all the peanut sauce ingredients, except the hot water, in a small blender and blend until smooth. Add hot water, 1 tablespoon at a time, until your desired consistency is reached. The peanut sauce should be pourable, but not too thin and watery. Taste and adjust the seasonings, if needed.

FOR THE SALAD: Preheat the oven to 220°C/425°F/gas mark 7. Line a baking tray with a silicone mat or baking parchment.

Spread out the sweet potato slices in a single layer on the prepared tray and bake until softened and slightly browned, about 20 minutes. Set aside.

While the sweet potato is roasting, bring a saucepan of water fitted with a steamer basket to the boil over a medium-high heat. Add the green beans and carrots and steam until just tender, about 3 minutes. Transfer the green beans and carrots to a bowl of ice water to stop the cooking process. Drain and set aside.

TO SERVE: Spread the shredded lettuce in a large shallow bowl or on a platter. In separate piles, top the lettuce with all of the cooked and raw vegetables, as well as the tempeh, in this order: roasted sweet potato, steamed green beans, steamed carrots, sliced cucumber, sliced red bell pepper, bean sprouts, steamed tempeh and coriander. Ladle some of the peanut sauce over the dish, sprinkle on the peanuts, and serve the remaining sauce on the side.

3

PASTA

We don't have to say *basta* to pasta. True, bread collapses into a slurry of starch that is rapidly absorbed,[40] but the compact structure of pasta caused by the high-pressure compression during production slows down digestion,[41] so there's no need to completely deflour our diet. Is some pasta better than others? Whole-grain pasta leaves people feeling fuller compared to refined-grain pasta,[42] and 'pasta' made from vegetables, such as spiralized courgettes and spaghetti squash noodles, gives you all the heart and weight-loss benefits of veggies in a pasta-like form. *Mangia! Mangia!*

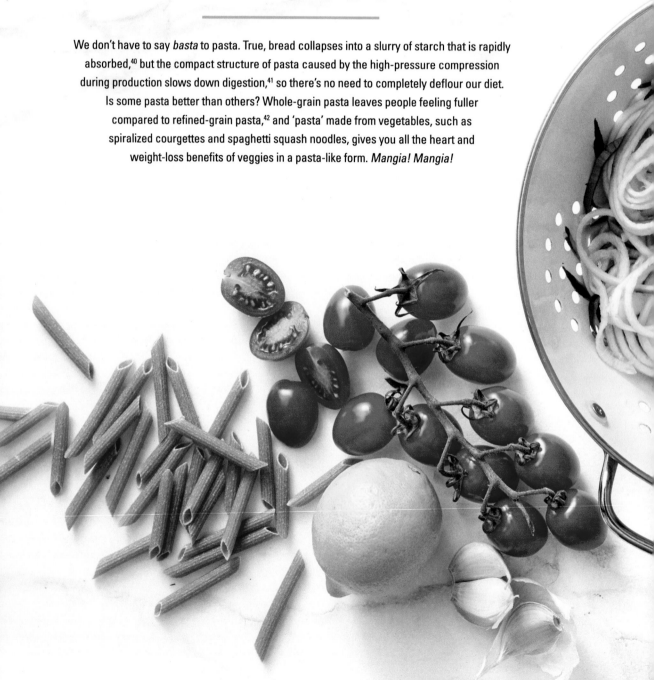

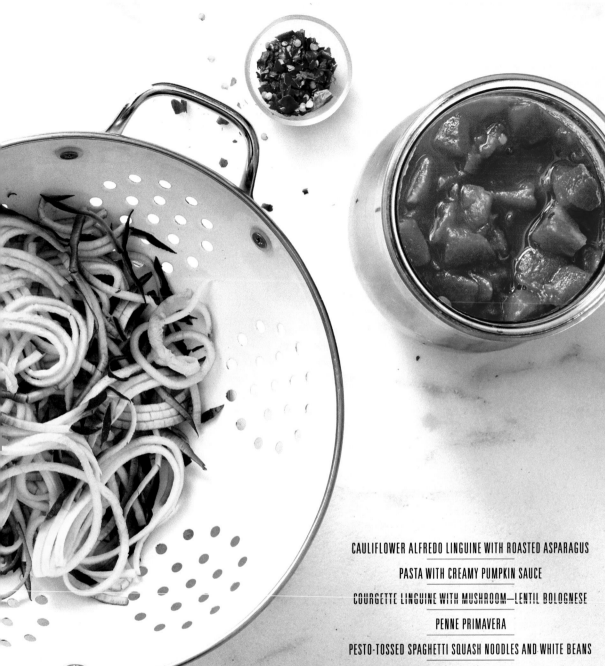

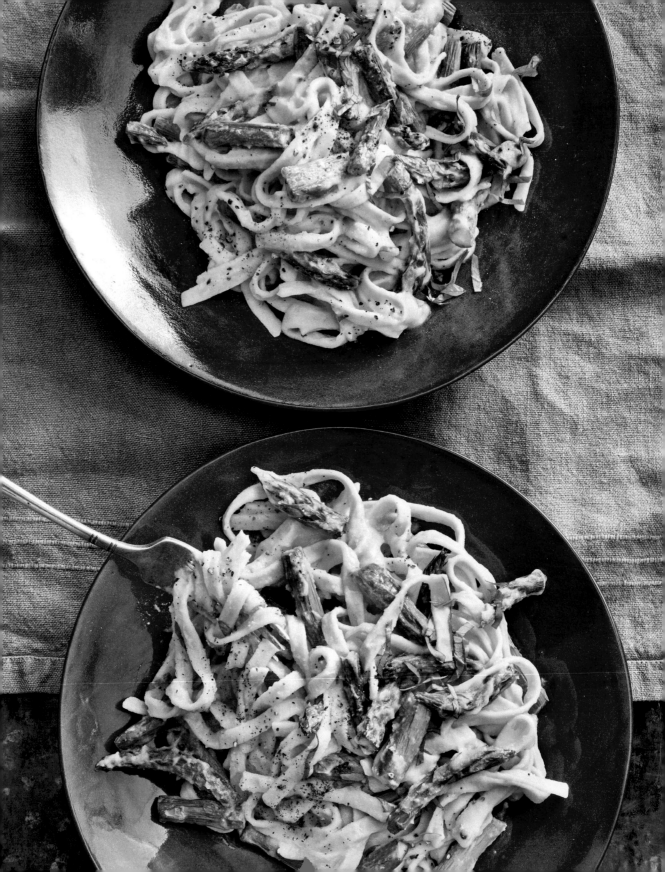

CAULIFLOWER ALFREDO LINGUINE WITH ROASTED ASPARAGUS

MAKES: *4 servings*   DIFFICULTY: *Easy*

Cauliflower is so versatile, delicious whether roasted, riced, pureed, steamed, water-sautéed or enjoyed raw. This amazing-for-you crucifer works its magic to make this creamy Alfredo sauce that tastes so decadent.

ALFREDO SAUCE

½ cup/75g chopped onion, or 2 large shallots, chopped

3 garlic cloves, finely chopped

1 head cauliflower, cored and chopped (3 to 4 cups/375 to 500g)

1 cup/250ml Light Vegetable Broth (page 214)

2 tablespoons nutritional yeast

1 tablespoon white miso paste

½ tablespoon fresh lemon juice

ASPARAGUS

1 pound/450g asparagus, trimmed and cut into 1½-inch/4cm pieces

LINGUINE

8 ounces/225g whole-grain or bean-based linguine

TO SERVE

Brazil Nut Parm (page 210)

2 tablespoons chopped fresh basil

Coarsely ground black pepper

FOR THE ALFREDO SAUCE: Heat ¼ cup/60ml of water in a large saucepan over a medium-high heat. Add the onion and cook for 4 minutes to soften. Add the garlic and cook for 30 seconds. Add the cauliflower and Light Vegetable Broth and bring to the boil. Lower the heat to a simmer, cover, and cook for about 12 minutes, or until the cauliflower is soft.

Transfer the cauliflower mixture to a high-powered blender and blend on high speed until smooth. Add the nutritional yeast, miso paste, and lemon juice and blend until smooth and creamy. Pour the sauce into a saucepan and keep warm over a very low heat.

FOR THE ASPARAGUS: Preheat the oven to 220°C/425°F/gas mark 7. Line a rimmed baking tray with a silicone mat or baking parchment.

Arrange the asparagus in a single layer on the prepared tray. Roast in the oven for 15 minutes, or until the asparagus is tender and slightly browned.

FOR THE LINGUINE: Cook the linguine according to the package instructions in a pot of boiling water, stirring occasionally, until al dente. Drain the pasta and return it to the pot. Add the roasted asparagus and Alfredo sauce and heat for a few minutes until hot, tossing gently to combine.

TO SERVE: Divide the pasta among shallow serving bowls or plates and serve hot, topped with the Brazil Nut Parm to taste, basil, and black pepper to taste.

PASTA WITH CREAMY PUMPKIN SAUCE

MAKES: *4 servings*   DIFFICULTY: *Easy*

This creamy pasta dish is especially welcome on cold autumn nights. Use your favourite whole-grain or bean-based pasta shape. Consider serving the sauce over black bean pasta for Halloween!

½ cup/125ml Light Vegetable Broth (page 214)

1 onion, chopped

3 garlic cloves, finely chopped

1 teaspoon garlic powder

1 teaspoon onion powder

½ teaspoon dried oregano

½ teaspoon dried basil

¼ teaspoon red pepper flakes

1 (400g) BPA-free tin solid-pack pumpkin puree (*not* pumpkin pie filling)

1 (400g) BPA-free tin or Tetra Pak salt-free finely chopped tomatoes

2 tablespoons nutritional yeast

2 teaspoons white miso paste

2 teaspoons balsamic vinegar

Ground black pepper

8 ounces/225g whole-grain or bean-based pasta of choice

Chopped fresh parsley

Brazil Nut Parm (page 210) (optional)

Heat the Light Vegetable Broth in a saucepan over a medium heat. Add the onion and garlic and cook, stirring frequently, until the onion is soft, 5 to 7 minutes. Add the garlic powder, onion powder, oregano, basil and red pepper flakes. Stir in the pumpkin puree and finely chopped tomatoes and cook, stirring, for about 10 minutes. Taste and adjust the seasonings as desired. Remove from the heat.

Carefully transfer the pumpkin mixture to a blender. Add the nutritional yeast, miso paste, vinegar and black pepper to taste. Blend until smooth and creamy. If the sauce is too thick, add a little more Light Vegetable Broth or water. Set aside.

Cook the pasta according to the package instructions in a pot of oiling water until al dente. Drain the pasta and return it to the pot. Add as much of the sauce as desired, tossing gently to coat the pasta, and heat the sauce. Serve hot, topped with fresh parsley and Brazil Nut Parm (if using).

GARLIC POWDER AND HEART DISEASE

Heart disease patients got a 50 per cent increase in artery function with only a daily ¼ teaspoon of garlic powder,[43] which may be considered as an adjunct treatment for atherosclerosis, our number one killer.[44] Garlic also has a significant beneficial effect on blood pressure.[45]

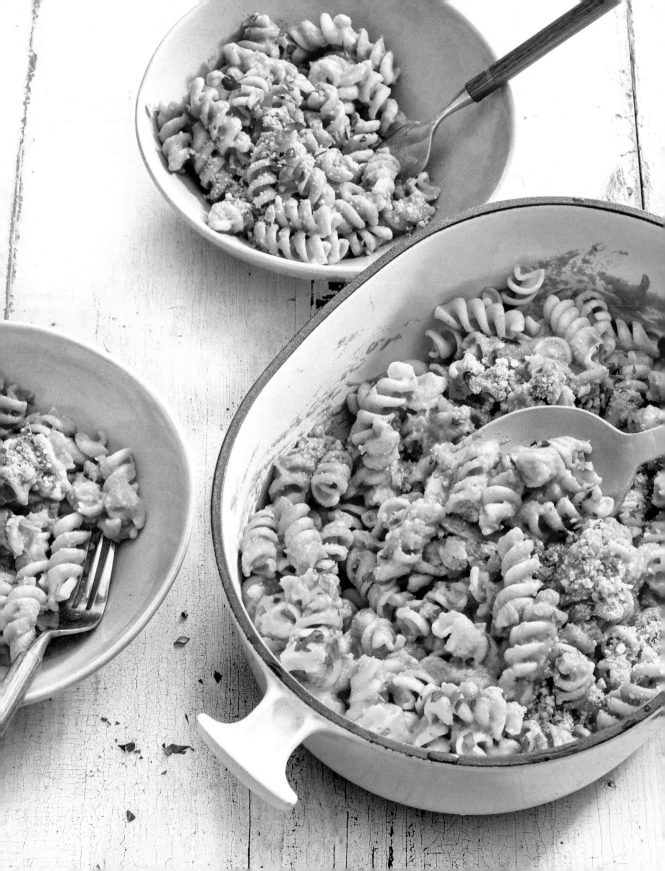

COURGETTE LINGUINE WITH MUSHROOM-LENTIL BOLOGNESE

MAKES: *4 servings*   DIFFICULTY: *Moderate*

If you've never made your own courgette noodles, you may be surprised how easy it is. Simply cut the squash into long, thin strips, using a mandoline slicer, sharp knife or a peeler, or just use a spiralizer, if you have one. The squash strips should resemble strands of pasta. If you don't have time to make your own, look for packages of already spiralized courgette noodles in the produce section of your supermarket. You can also substitute 8 ounces/225g of whole-grain or bean-based linguine, if you prefer. I use black lentils in the sauce, but you can use any type of lentils you have on hand.

BOLOGNESE SAUCE
¾ cup/150g dried black lentils

1 onion, finely chopped

3 garlic cloves, finely chopped

8 ounces/225g baby portobello mushrooms, finely chopped

3 tablespoons salt-free tomato puree

1 tablespoon white miso paste

2 tablespoons nutritional yeast

½ teaspoon dried oregano

½ teaspoon dried basil

¼ teaspoon red pepper flakes (optional)

2 (400g) BPA-free tins or Tetra Paks salt-free finely chopped tomatoes

1 teaspoon balsamic vinegar

COURGETTE NOODLES
4 to 6 courgettes, trimmed and spiralized or cut into long, thin strips to resemble noodles

TO SERVE
Brazil Nut Parm (page 210)

FOR THE BOLOGNESE SAUCE: Cook* the lentils in a pressure cooker or a pot on the stovetop. Set aside.

Heat ¼ cup/60ml of water in a large, deep skillet or saucepan over a medium heat. Add the onion and garlic and cook, stirring occasionally, until softened, about 5 minutes. Add the mushrooms and cook for 3 minutes longer, and then stir in the tomato puree, miso paste, nutritional yeast, oregano, basil and red pepper flakes (if using). Add the tomatoes and cooked lentils and simmer, stirring frequently, for 15 minutes or until the sauce has thickened and the flavours have blended. Stir in the vinegar and then taste and adjust the seasonings, if needed. Keep warm over a low heat.

FOR THE COURGETTE NOODLES: While the sauce is simmering, cook the courgette noodles in a large pot of boiling water, stirring occasionally, until they are just tender, 3 to 5 minutes. Drain and set aside.

TO SERVE: Divide the cooked courgette noodles among shallow serving bowls or plates and top with the sauce. Sprinkle with Brazil Nut Parm to taste and serve hot.

Turn to the Legumes and Grains Cooking Charts *on pages 218–221 for instruction, if needed.*

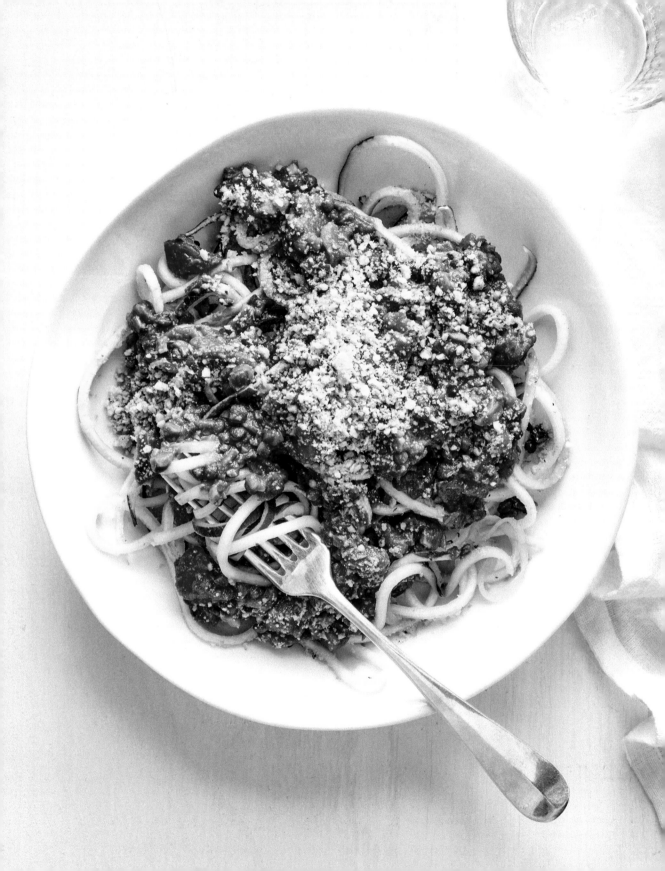

PENNE PRIMAVERA

MAKES: *4 servings*   DIFFICULTY: *Easy*

When you see 'primavera', you know there will be a lot of vegetables. This take on a classic features veggies tossed with whole-grain pasta and a creamy white bean sauce. *Buon appetito!*

1 cup/175g cooked* or BPA-free tinned or Tetra Pak salt-free white beans, drained and rinsed

1 cup/250ml Light Vegetable Broth (page 214)

3 tablespoons nutritional yeast

2 teaspoons miso paste

1 teaspoon balsamic vinegar

1 teaspoon fresh lemon juice

1 teaspoon onion powder

½ teaspoon garlic powder

1½ teaspoons dried basil

½ teaspoon dried marjoram

Ground black pepper

8 ounces/225g whole-grain or bean-based penne or other bite-size pasta of choice

1½ cups/100g small broccoli florets

1 carrot, thinly sliced

1 small courgette or yellow squash, cut into ¼-inch/5mm dice

2 spring onions, chopped

1 cup/150g cherry tomatoes, halved lengthways

2 tablespoons Brazil Nut Parm (page 210)

2 tablespoons chopped fresh basil or flat-leaf parsley

In a high-powered blender or food processor, combine the white beans, Light Vegetable Broth, nutritional yeast, miso paste, vinegar, lemon juice, onion powder, garlic powder, basil, marjoram and black pepper to taste. Blend until smooth. Taste and adjust the seasonings, if needed. Set the sauce aside.

Cook the penne according to the packet instructions in a large pot of boiling water, stirring occasionally, until it is tender, about 10 minutes. About 5 minutes before the pasta is cooked, add the broccoli and carrots. About 2 minutes before the pasta is cooked, add the courgette. Drain the cooked pasta and vegetables and return them to the pot. Add the sauce, spring onions and tomatoes and cook over a medium-low heat for a few minutes, tossing gently to heat through and coat the pasta and veggies with the sauce. Serve hot, sprinkled with the Brazil Nut Parm and fresh basil or parsley.

*Turn to the Legumes and Grains Cooking Charts *on pages 218–221 for instruction, if needed.*

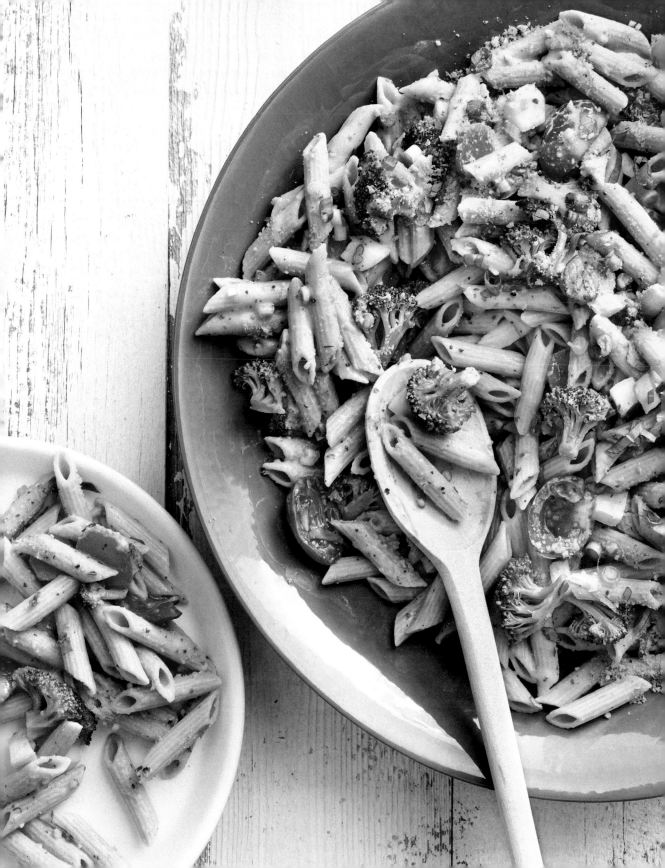

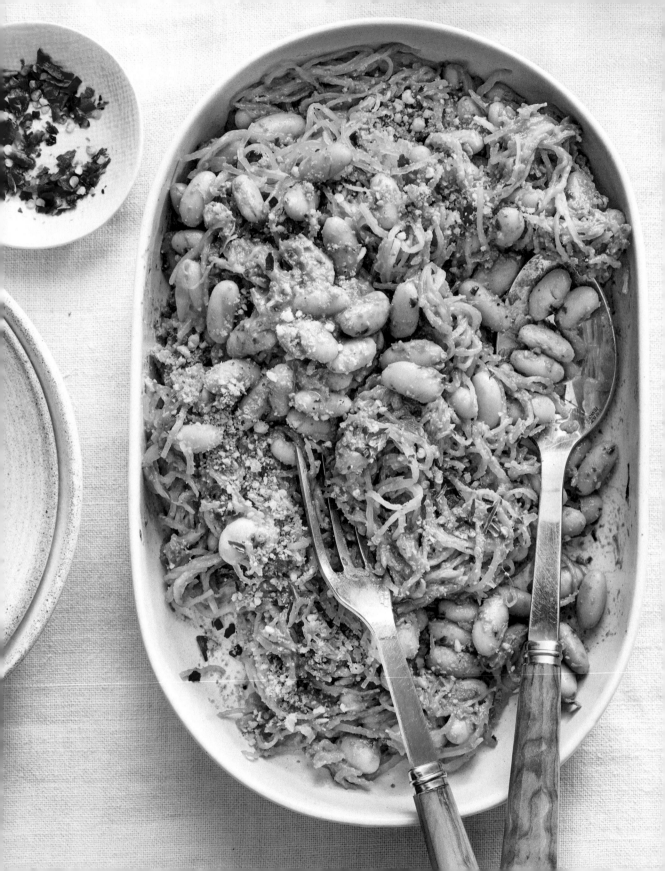

PESTO-TOSSED SPAGHETTI SQUASH NOODLES AND WHITE BEANS

MAKES: *4 servings*   DIFFICULTY: *Easy*

The fragrant Basil Pesto and cooked white beans add a deep flavour and interesting texture to baked spaghetti squash and are delicious with cooked courgette noodles and whole-grain pasta, too.

1 large spaghetti squash, halved crosswise

1½ cups/375ml Basil Pesto (page 215)

1 cup/175g cooked* or BPA-free tinned or Tetra Pak salt-free white beans, drained and rinsed

Brazil Nut Parm (page 210)

¼ to ½ teaspoon red pepper flakes (optional)

IN THE OVEN: Preheat the oven to 200°C/400°F/gas mark 6. Place the squash halves, cut side up, in a baking dish. Add about an inch/2.5cm of water and cover the dish tightly with a lid. Bake until tender, 45 minutes to 1 hour.

When the squash is done baking, remove and discard its seeds, and then use a fork to scrape the squash into strands and place them in a large bowl.

IN A MULTICOOKER, SUCH AS AN INSTANT POT: Set a steamer basket or metal trivet in the bottom of the pot. Pour 1 cup/250ml of water into the bottom of the pot. Place the squash halves on the basket and secure the lid of the multicooker. Set the multicooker to cook for 8 minutes on high pressure. Use Quick Release and then carefully remove the squash. Allow the squash to cool for 10 minutes before removing the seeds and shredding the flesh.

TO SERVE: Add the Basil Pesto and white beans and toss gently to combine. Serve sprinkled with Brazil Nut Parm and red pepper flakes (if using).

Turn to the Legumes and Grains Cooking Charts *on pages 218–221 for instruction, if needed.*

PASTA WITH ROASTED TOMATO SAUCE

MAKES: *4 servings*   DIFFICULTY: *Easy*

Sometimes simplest is best. This easy-to-make tomato sauce has a rich depth of flavour, owing to the slow-roasting. Try to find large plum tomatoes for the sauce as they are less watery than other varieties. This sauce is delicious over any type of pasta.

ROASTED TOMATO SAUCE

2 pounds/450g ripe plum tomatoes, cored and halved

½ small red onion, chopped

3 garlic cloves, finely chopped

1 tablespoon Italian seasoning

Ground black pepper

PASTA

8 ounces/225g whole-grain or bean-based pasta of choice

2 tablespoons chopped fresh basil finely chopped fresh parsley

Brazil Nut Parm (page 210)

FOR THE ROASTED TOMATO SAUCE: Preheat the oven to 160°C/325°F/gas mark 3. Line a large, rimmed baking tray with a silicone mat or baking parchment.

Place the tomato halves, cut side up, in the prepared baking tray. Sprinkle with the onion, garlic, Italian seasoning and black pepper to taste. Roast in the oven for about 2 hours, or until the tomatoes begin to break down and release their juices. If you prefer a richer-tasting sauce, leave the tomatoes in the oven for an additional 30 to 45 minutes, or until caramelized.

Remove the tray from the oven and transfer the tomato mixture to a food processor. Process until the tomato sauce reaches the consistency you prefer. Transfer the sauce to a saucepan and heat over a low heat until hot. Taste and adjust the seasonings, if needed.

FOR THE PASTA: Cook the pasta according to the package instructions in a pot of boiling water until al dente. Drain and return the pasta to the pot. Add as much of the sauce as desired, tossing gently to coat the pasta, and heat the sauce. Serve hot, topped with basil or parsley and Brazil Nut Parm.

TOMATO SAUCE FOR PROSTATE CANCER

What about tomatoes versus lycopene, their antioxidant red pigment, and prostate cancer? A tomato sauce-based intervention decreased PSA concentrations in prostate cancer patients and free radical damage of their DNA.[46] The whole may be more powerful than its parts when it comes to whole fruits and vegetables, compared to supplementing with an isolated single compound.

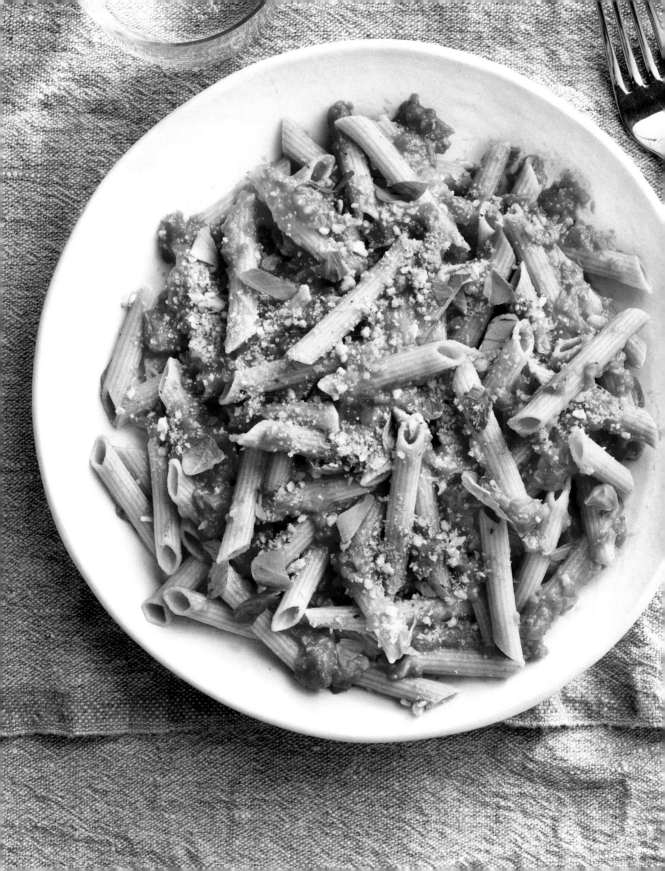

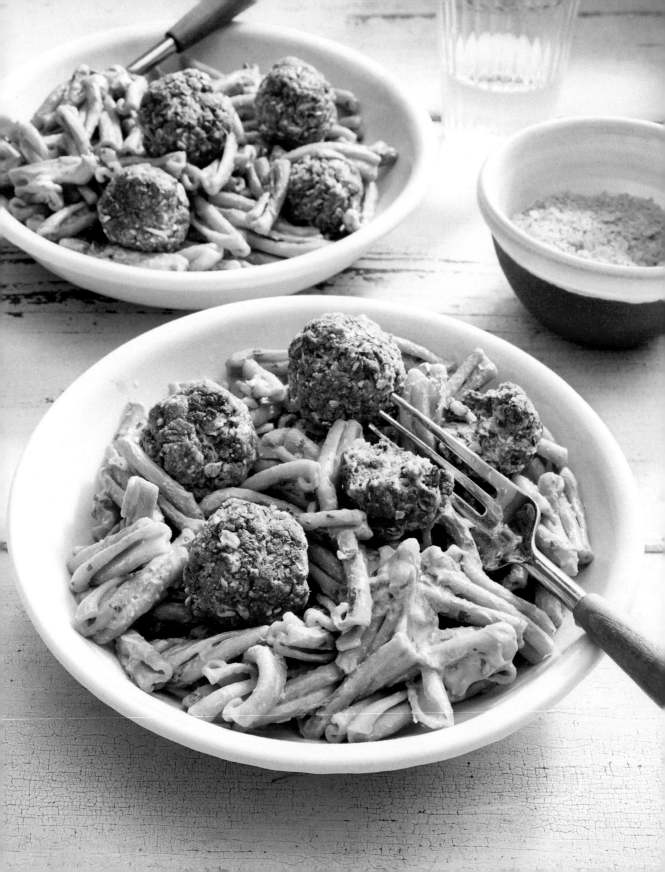

GEMELLI WITH COURGETTE MEATBALLS AND CHIMICHURRI

MAKES: *4 servings*   DIFFICULTY: *Moderate*

Don't let this recipe's length intimidate you. It's as simple to make as it is delicious. I like to make the meatballs and sauce ahead of time so their flavours develop even more. When I'm not in the mood for chimichurri sauce, I substitute my favourite salt-free marinara or the Roasted Tomato Sauce on page 80.

COURGETTE MEATBALLS

1 (400g) BPA-free tin or Tetra Pak salt-free chickpeas, drained, rinsed, and blotted dry

3 garlic cloves, smashed

⅓ cup/35g old-fashioned rolled oats

3 tablespoons nutritional yeast

3 tablespoons ground flaxseeds

1 tablespoon ground chia seeds

2 teaspoons fresh lemon juice

1 teaspoon white miso paste

1½ teaspoons dried basil

1½ teaspoons dried oregano

1 teaspoon onion powder

¼ teaspoon ground black pepper

1 cup/150g grated courgette, squeezed dry

CHIMICHURRI SAUCE

2 ripe Hass avocados, peeled and pitted

2 tablespoons fresh lemon juice

1 tablespoon red wine vinegar

2 to 3 garlic cloves, finely chopped

1 teaspoon white miso paste

½ teaspoon dried oregano

¼ teaspoon red pepper flakes, or to taste

¼ teaspoon ground black pepper

¼ cup/4 tablespoons chopped fresh coriander

¼ cup/4 tablespoons chopped fresh parsley

PASTA

8 ounces/225g whole-grain or bean-based gemelli or other pasta of choice

FOR THE COURGETTE MEATBALLS: Combine the chickpeas, garlic, oats, nutritional yeast, flaxseeds and chia seeds in a food processor and pulse until finely chopped. Add the lemon juice, miso paste, basil, oregano, onion powder and black pepper. Pulse until thoroughly mixed. Transfer to a large bowl and add the grated courgette. Stir together until well combined. The mixture should hold together when pinched between two fingers. If the mixture is too wet, add a little nutritional yeast or ground flaxseeds to absorb excess moisture.

Preheat the oven to 190°C/375°F/gas mark 5. Line a baking tray with a silicone mat or baking parchment.

Scoop about 2 tablespoons of the courgette mixture at a time and use your hands to roll the mixture into balls. Arrange the courgette balls on the prepared baking tray and bake for 25 minutes, or until firm and lightly browned.

FOR THE CHIMICHURRI SAUCE: In a food processor, combine all the chimichurri sauce ingredients plus ¼ cup/60ml of water and pulse to combine. Set aside.

FOR THE PASTA: Cook the pasta according to the packet instructions in a pot of boiling water until al dente. Drain and return to the pot. Add the chimichurri sauce and toss gently to combine. Divide the pasta into shallow serving bowls and top each portion with 3 or 4 courgette meatballs.

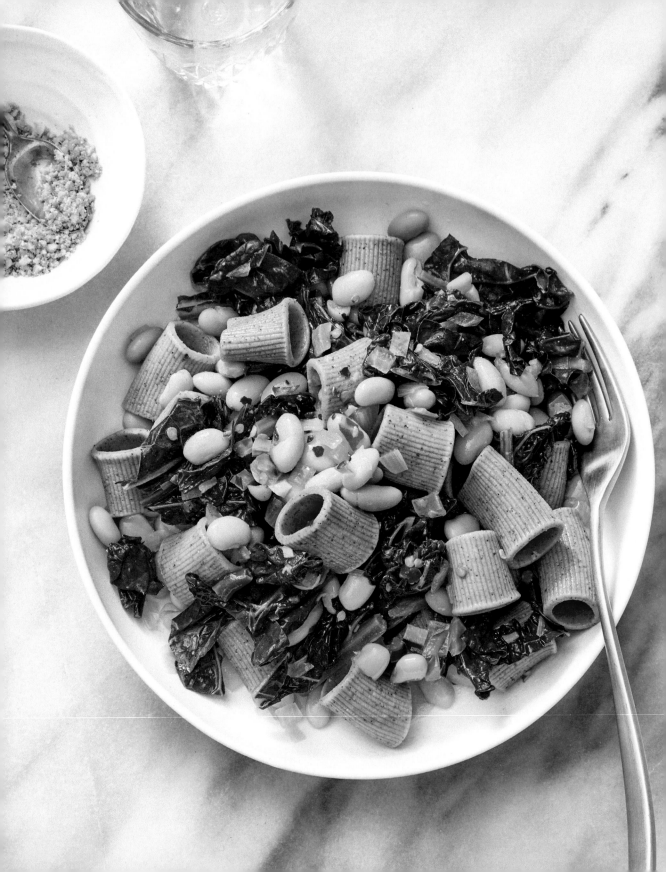

PASTA WITH GARLICKY WHITE BEANS AND CAVOLO NERO

MAKES: *4 to 6 servings*   DIFFICULTY: *Easy*

Many Italian dishes combine greens and beans – and pasta, of course! This one is made with cavolo nero (Italian kale), but you can substitute any dark leafy greens you desire.

½ cup/75g finely chopped red onion

3 garlic cloves, finely chopped

½ cup/125ml Light Vegetable Broth (page 214)

3 tablespoons nutritional yeast

1 tablespoon white miso paste

½ teaspoon garlic powder

¼ teaspoon red pepper flakes

1 pound/450g cavolo nero, trimmed and cut crossways into 1-inch/2.5cm slices

3 cups/525g cooked* or 2 (400g) BPA-free tins or Tetra Paks salt-free cannellini beans or white beans, drained and rinsed

Ground black pepper

1 tablespoon white balsamic vinegar

8 ounces/225g whole-grain or bean-based pasta of choice

Heat ¼ cup/60ml of water in a large saucepan or deep skillet over a medium-high heat. Add the onion and garlic and cook until the onion is soft, about 7 minutes. Lower the heat to a simmer and stir in the Light Vegetable Broth, nutritional yeast, miso paste, garlic powder and red pepper flakes. Add the cavolo nero and cook, stirring occasionally, until it is wilted, about 2 minutes. Add the white beans and black pepper to taste. Cover and cook until the cavolo nero is tender, about 10 minutes. Stir in the vinegar and then taste and adjust the seasonings, if needed. Keep warm.

While the cavolo nero and beans are simmering, cook the pasta according to the packet instructions in a large pot of boiling water, stirring occasionally, until al dente. Drain well and return to the pot. Add the cavolo nero mixture and toss gently to combine. Serve hot.

Turn to the Legumes and Grains Cooking Charts *on pages 218–221 for instruction, if needed.*

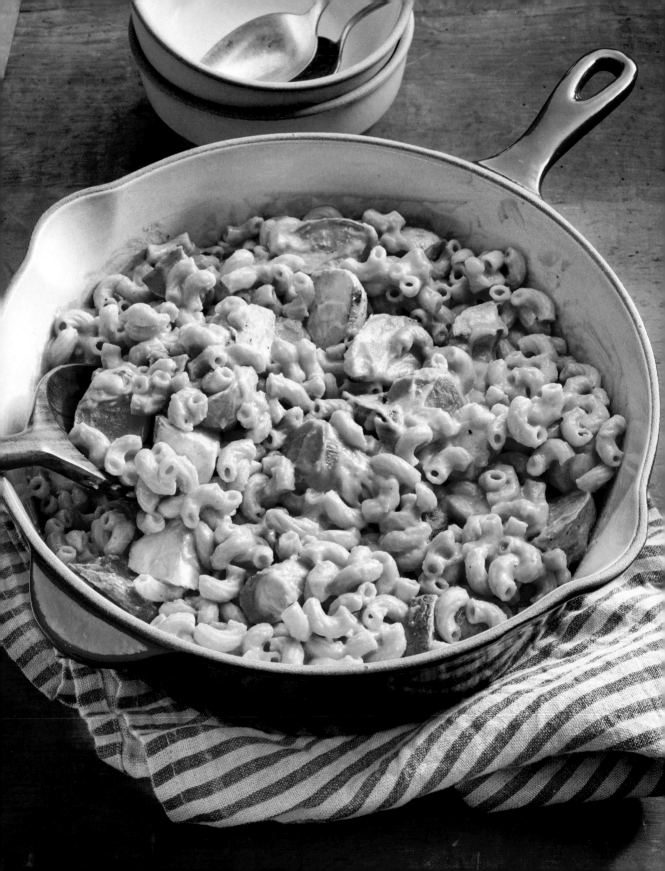

ROOT VEGETABLE MAC 'N CHEESE

MAKES: *4 servings*   DIFFICULTY: *Moderate*

Root vegetable lovers rejoice! This dish not only features chunks of roasted root vegetables, but there are pureed root veggies in the sauce, too. Follow the recipe closely, or use your own combination of root vegetables, including swede and celery (though you may want to avoid beetroot unless you want pink mac 'n cheese). You will need about 3 pounds/1.35kg in total.

ROOT VEGETABLES

1 parsnip, cut into 1-inch/2.5cm dice

1 carrot, cut into 1-inch/2.5cm dice

1 sweet potato, cut into 1-inch/2.5cm dice

1 waxy potato, cut into 1-inch/2.5cm dice

½ cup/75g chopped onion

½ teaspoon onion powder

¼ teaspoon ground black pepper

MAC 'N CHEESE

2 cups/500ml Light Vegetable Broth (page 214), or more as needed

½ cup/70g nutritional yeast

1 tablespoon fresh lemon juice

1 teaspoon white miso paste

1 teaspoon salt-free mustard

½ teaspoon onion powder

½ teaspoon garlic powder

½ teaspoon smoked paprika

¼ teaspoon grated fresh turmeric, or ¼ teaspoon ground

8 ounces/225g whole-grain or bean-based elbow macaroni or other bite-size pasta of your choice

FOR THE ROOT VEGETABLES: Preheat the oven to 220°C/425°F/gas mark 7. Line two baking trays with silicone mats or baking parchment.

Divide the vegetables evenly in a single layer between the two prepared trays. Sprinkle with onion powder and black pepper. Roast until the vegetables are tender and slightly caramelized, 45 to 60 minutes, turning the veggies with a metal spatula about halfway through. When the vegetables are done roasting, remove them from the oven and set aside.

FOR THE MAC 'N CHEESE: Put 2 cups/350g of the roasted vegetables into a high-powered blender. Add the Light Vegetable Broth, nutritional yeast, lemon juice, miso paste, mustard, onion powder, garlic powder, paprika and turmeric. Blend until very smooth. Taste and adjust the seasonings, if necessary. Add more broth if needed to reach your desired consistency. Set the sauce aside.

Cook the macaroni according to the packet instructions in a large pot of boiling water until al dente. Drain well and return to the pot. Add the remaining roasted vegetables and the sauce, stirring gently over a low heat to combine and heat through. Serve hot.

THE BEST WAY TO COOK FOR OUR EYES AND BRAIN

Lutein, the antioxidant in green vegetables,[47] protects our light-sensing nerves, helping us see better[48] and perhaps think better.[49] Boiling increases lutein levels,[50] whereas microwaving may be detrimental. The best? Steaming, which nearly doubles lutein levels.[51]

GREEN BEAN AND MUSHROOM STROGANOFF

MAKES: *4 servings*   DIFFICULTY: *Moderate*

There are so many reasons I love this dish, including its versatility. If you're not in the mood for green beans, for example, you can substitute different vegetables, such as peppers and courgettes. Instead of mushrooms, use diced braised tempeh, or go the other way and add even more 'shrooms. Rather than serving over pasta, spoon the savoury Stroganoff over cooked greens or whole grains. Innovate and create!

8 ounces/225g green beans, trimmed and cut into 1.5-inch/4cm pieces

1 cup/250ml Light Vegetable Broth (page 214)

1 onion, chopped

3 garlic cloves, finely chopped

1 pound/450g baby portobello mushrooms, trimmed and quartered

1 teaspoon dried thyme

¼ teaspoon ground black pepper

1 cup/175g cooked* or BPA-free tinned or Tetra Pak salt-free white beans, drained and rinsed

3 tablespoons nutritional yeast

2 teaspoons fresh lemon juice

2 teaspoons white miso paste

8 ounces/225g whole-grain or bean-based linguine

⅓ cup/20g chopped fresh parsley

Place a steamer basket in a pot with about 1 inch/2.5cm of water. Add the green beans and steam over boiling water until just tender, about 4 minutes. Set aside.

Heat the Light Vegetable Broth in a large saucepan over a medium heat. Add the onion and garlic and cook until the onion is tender, about 5 minutes. Stir in the mushrooms, thyme and black pepper. Continue to cook for another 5 minutes, or until the mushrooms have softened and begin to release their juices. Set the Stroganoff aside.

In a blender or food processor, combine the white beans, nutritional yeast, lemon juice, miso paste and ¼ cup/60ml of water. Blend until smooth. Scoop out 1 cup/250ml of the Stroganoff and add it to the bean mixture. Blend until smooth. If the sauce is too thick, add a little more water. If it is too thin, add more beans.

Stir the blended bean mixture into the saucepan containing the remaining Stroganoff. Add the steamed green beans, stirring to combine and heat through. Taste and adjust the seasonings, if needed. Keep warm over a low heat.

Cook the pasta according to the packet instructions in a pot of boiling water until al dente. Drain well, and then divide the noodles among shallow bowls. Top the noodles with the Stroganoff and sprinkle with fresh parsley. Serve hot.

*Turn to the Legumes and Grains Cooking Charts *on pages 218–221 for instruction, if needed.*

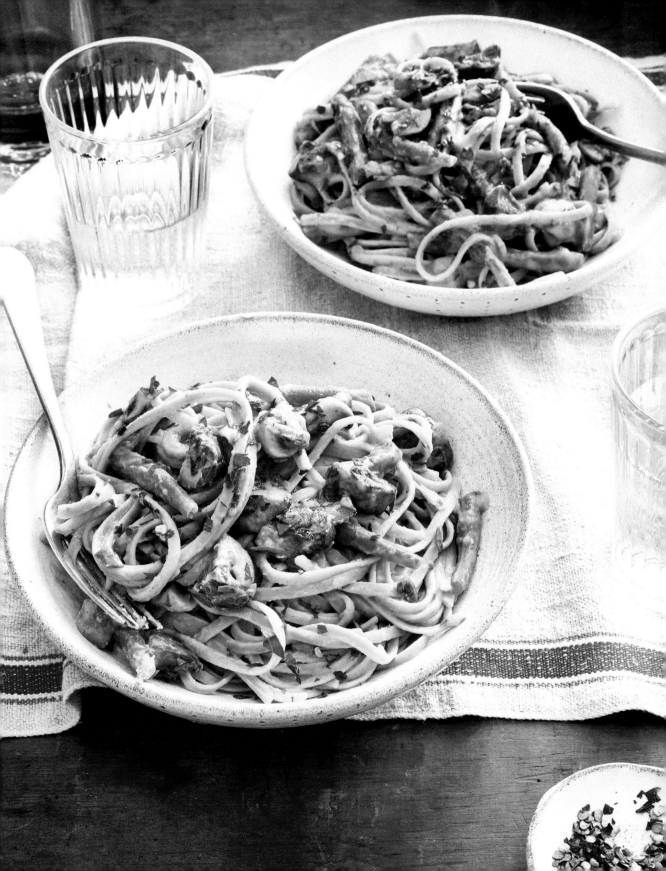

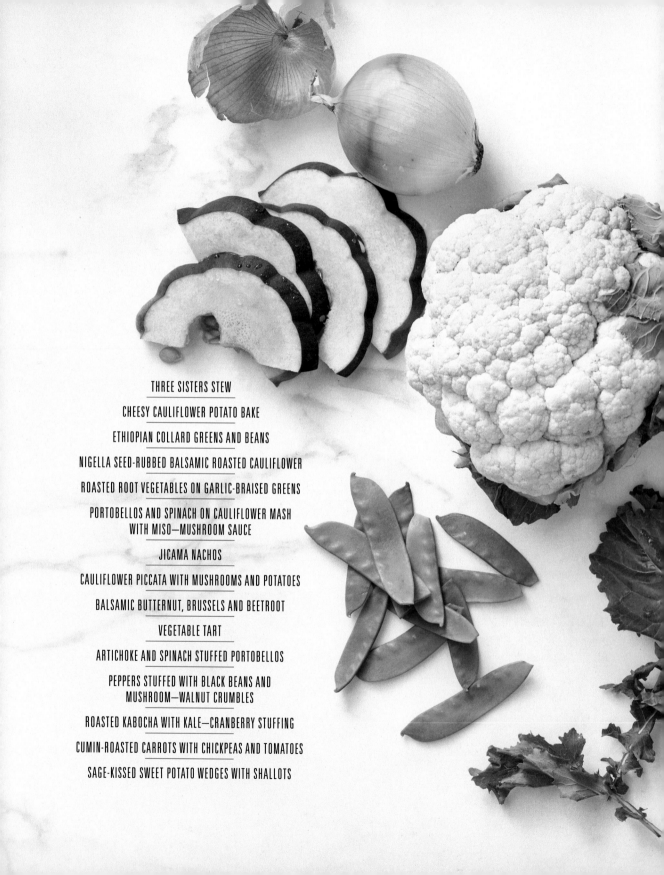

4

MAIN-LY VEGETABLES

Many vegetables have such a low calorie density that you would tire from chewing before you could overdo it. You'd have to eat a wheelbarrow full of cabbage before you'd ever need to begin worrying about overindulging. And the more water-rich the food, the fewer calories are being taken in overall. Higher-volume foods also take longer to eat, which slows the rate of consumption and increases 'oropharyngeal stimulation',[52] the sensation of food in our mouth and throat. The more we chew, taste, and feel food in our mouth, the more our brain gets tipped off that we're filling up.

Which foods have the most water? Vegetables top the charts, with most being more than 90 per cent water by weight, followed by most fruit coming in around the 80s. And, since all the calories in whole plant foods are not only trapped inside cells but are also inside cell walls made out of indigestible fibre, we end up with fewer calories in our system.[53] If these aren't enough reasons to get you to eat your veggies, these main-ly vegetable recipes are just too good to resist.

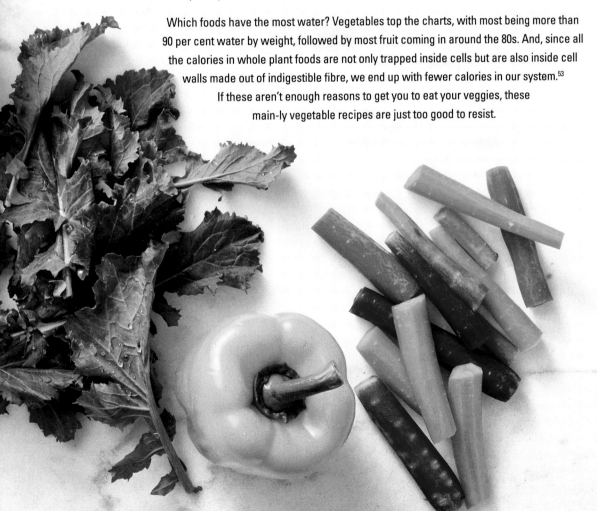

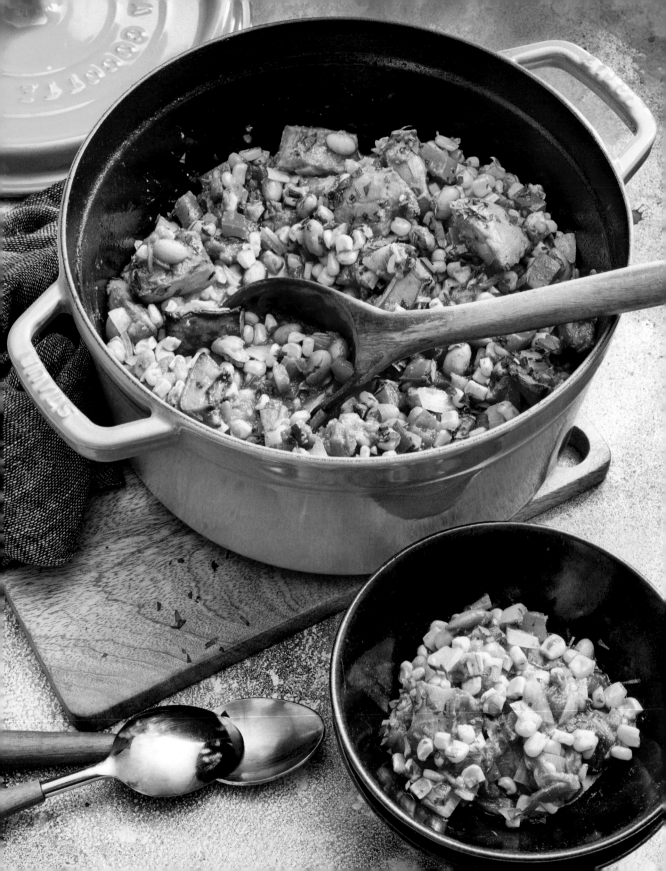

THREE SISTERS STEW

MAKES: *6 servings*   DIFFICULTY: *Easy*

According to Native American tradition, beans, corn and squash are the 'three sisters', planted together to support one other and allowing each to thrive. If you don't have time to dice your own squash, look for pre-diced squash in the produce section of your supermarket.

1 large butternut squash (about 2 pounds/900g), halved lengthways

½ teaspoon onion powder

½ teaspoon smoked paprika

1 cup/250ml Light Vegetable Broth (page 214) or water

1 onion, chopped

3 garlic cloves, finely chopped

1 large red pepper, cut into ½-inch/1cm dice

1 small fresh hot chilli, de-seeded and finely chopped or 1 (113g) BPA-free tin salt-free chopped mild green chillies, drained

1 (400g) BPA-free tin or Tetra Pak salt-free chopped tomatoes, undrained

3 cups/500g cooked* or 2 (400g) BPA-free tins or Tetra Paks salt-free pinto beans, drained and rinsed

2 cups/350g fresh or frozen sweetcorn

2 teaspoons ground cumin

2 teaspoons chilli powder

1 teaspoon dried oregano

Super-Charged Spice Blend (page 211)

Ground black pepper

¼ cup/4 tablespoons finely chopped fresh coriander or parsley

Preheat the oven to 190°C/375°F/gas mark 5. Line a rimmed baking tray with a silicone mat or baking parchment.

Scrape out the seeds and fibres from the squash, then cut the squash into 1½-inch/4cm dice. Evenly spread the diced squash in a single layer on the prepared baking tray. Sprinkle with the onion powder and paprika; then roast in the oven for about 45 minutes, or until just tender but not completely soft. (You should be able to pierce through a piece of squash with a knife and get a little resistance.) Set aside.

Heat the Light Vegetable Broth in a large pot over a medium heat. Add the onion and cook until softened, about 5 minutes. Add the garlic, pepper and chilli and continue to cook until the vegetables are tender, about 5 minutes longer. Stir in the tomatoes with their liquid, pinto beans, sweetcorn, cumin, chilli powder and oregano. Season with Super-Charged Spice Blend and ground black pepper to taste. Add the roasted squash and bring to a simmer. Cover and simmer gently until all the vegetables are tender and the flavours have developed, about 20 minutes. The stew should be thick, but if it thickens too much, add a little more broth. Just before serving, stir in the coriander. Taste and adjust the seasonings, if needed. Serve hot.

Turn to the Legumes and Grains Cooking Charts on pages 218–221 for instruction, if needed.

CHEESY CAULIFLOWER POTATO BAKE

MAKES: *4 servings*   DIFFICULTY: *Easy*

A crisp green salad is the perfect accompaniment to this cozy casserole made with cauliflower, potatoes and white beans. For variation, add a layer of sliced tomatoes when assembling for a pop of colour and even more veggies. You can also make this with sliced sweet potatoes instead of floury ones, if you prefer, or use one of each.

1½ cups/260g cooked* or 1 (400g) BPA-free tin or Tetra Pak salt-free white beans, drained and rinsed

⅔ cup/90g nutritional yeast

1½ tablespoons fresh lemon juice

1 tablespoon apple cider vinegar

2 teaspoons white miso paste

1 teaspoon salt-free mustard

1 teaspoon onion powder

1 teaspoon dried thyme

1 (½-inch/1cm) piece fresh turmeric, grated, or ½ teaspoon ground

½ teaspoon garlic powder

Ground black pepper

2 cups/500ml Light Vegetable Broth (page 214)

1 head cauliflower, cored and cut into ¼-inch/5mm slices

2 floury potatoes, thinly sliced

¼ cup/25g finely ground walnuts

½ teaspoon smoked paprika

In a food processor or high-powered blender, combine the beans, nutritional yeast, lemon juice, apple cider vinegar, miso paste, mustard, onion powder, thyme, turmeric, garlic powder and black pepper to taste. Blend until very smooth. Add the Light Vegetable Broth and blend again. Taste and adjust the seasonings, if needed.

Preheat the oven to 200°C/400°F/gas mark 6.

Spread a thin layer of the sauce in the bottom of a large, shallow baking dish. Top the sauce with cauliflower slices so they evenly cover the dish in a single layer. Top the cauliflower slices with a layer of potato slices and then a layer of the sauce. Continue to layer with the remaining cauliflower and potatoes, ending with a layer of sauce on top.

Cover tightly and bake for 45 minutes. Remove from the oven and sprinkle the top with the ground walnuts and smoked paprika. Return the dish to the oven and bake, uncovered, until the vegetables are tender and the top is golden brown, about 15 minutes longer. Serve hot.

Turn to the Legumes and Grains Cooking Charts *on pages 218–221 for instruction, if needed.*

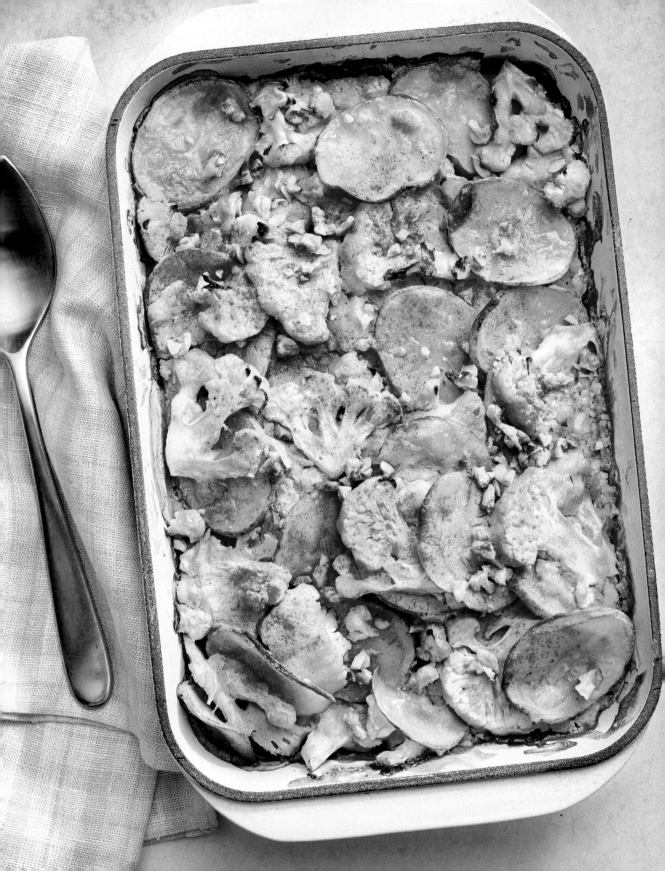

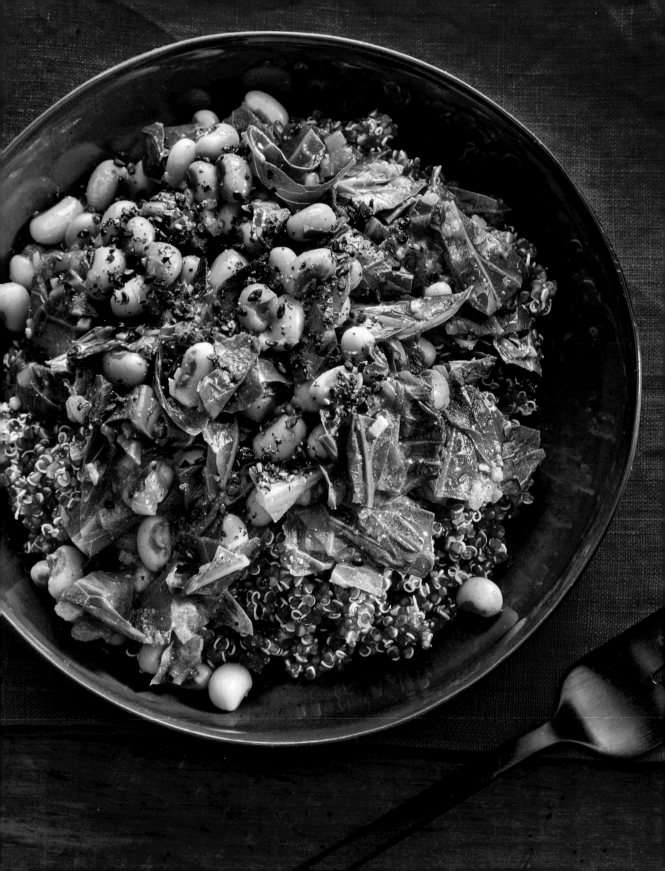

ETHIOPIAN COLLARD GREENS AND BEANS

MAKES: *4 servings*   DIFFICULTY: *Easy*

If you can't find fresh collard greens, kale is a good alternative, but keep in mind that the cooking time will be a bit shorter.

1 large red onion, finely chopped

3 garlic cloves, finely chopped

1½ teaspoons grated fresh ginger

1 teaspoon ground cumin

1 teaspoon ground coriander

1 teaspoon smoked paprika

½ teaspoon ground turmeric

¼ teaspoon ground fenugreek seeds

¼ teaspoon ground cardamom

¼ teaspoon cayenne, or more to taste

Super-Charged Spice Blend (page 211)

Ground black pepper

2 cups/500ml Light Vegetable Broth (page 214)

1 bunch collard greens (about 12 ounces/350g), thick stems removed, coarsely chopped

1½ cups/260g cooked* or 1 (400g) BPA-free tin or Tetra Pak salt-free black-eyed beans, drained and rinsed

White balsamic vinegar

Cooked* whole grains

¼ teaspoon coarsely ground nigella seeds

Heat ¼ cup/60ml of water in a large pot over a medium heat. Add the onion and cook for 5 minutes to soften. Add the garlic and ginger and cook, stirring, for 1 minute. Stir in the cumin, coriander, paprika, turmeric, fenugreek, cardamom and cayenne, and the Super-Charged Spice Blend and black pepper to taste. Add the Light Vegetable Broth and bring to the boil; then lower the heat to a simmer and add the collard greens, stirring until they wilt. Cover and cook for 30 minutes. Add the black-eyed beans and stir gently to combine. Continue to cook, uncovered, until the collards are tender and the liquid has mostly evaporated. When ready to serve, stir in a little vinegar, to taste. Spoon the greens over whole grains, sprinkle the nigella seeds on top, and serve hot.

＊*Turn to the* Legumes and Grains Cooking Charts *on pages 218–221 for instruction, if needed.*

BENEFITS OF FIBRE ON MORTALITY

Can fibre consumption influence cardiovascular, cancer and all-cause mortality? Those who ate the most fibre had 23 per cent less cardiovascular disease mortality, 17 per cent lower risk of dying from cancer, and 23 per cent lower mortality from all causes put together.[54]

Where is fibre found? Animal cells are encased only in easily digestible membranes, but the walls of plant cells are made out of fibre.

Looking for fibre? Look no further than whole, unrefined plant foods.[55]

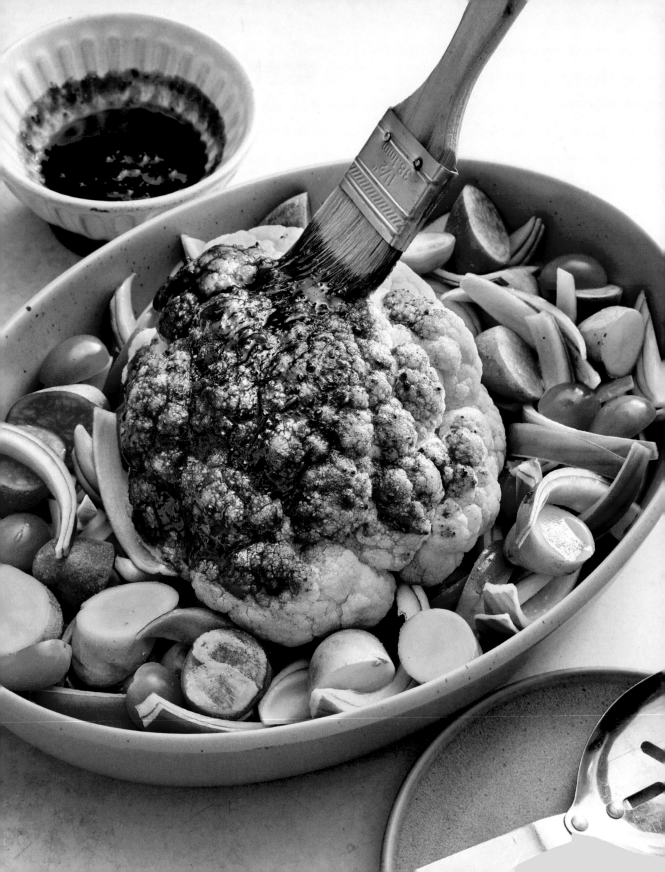

NIGELLA SEED-RUBBED BALSAMIC ROASTED CAULIFLOWER

MAKES: *4 servings*   DIFFICULTY: *Easy*

A whole, roasted cauliflower makes a great centrepiece on the dinner table, and this one, with its gorgeous dark bronze glaze, is just stunning.

1 cup/250ml balsamic vinegar

2 tablespoons Date Syrup (page 217)

2 teaspoons ground nigella seeds

1 large head cauliflower, cored, leaves removed

1 red onion, cut into ½-inch/1cm wedges

8 ounces/225g baby potatoes, halved

2 cups/300g cherry tomatoes, halved

2 tablespoons chopped fresh parsley

In a small saucepan over a medium heat, combine the vinegar, Date Syrup and 1 teaspoon of the ground nigella seeds. Bring to the boil, then lower the heat to low and simmer until reduced by half, about 20 minutes.

Preheat the oven to 200°C/400°F/gas mark 6. Line a large, shallow baking dish with a silicone mat or baking parchment.

While the balsamic mixture is simmering, pour about 3 inches/7.5cm of water into a pot large enough for the cauliflower head to sit upright and bring to the boil. Carefully place the cauliflower head upright in the boiling water. Cover and cook until lightly blanched, about 5 minutes. Use a large spatula to carefully remove it from the pot and transfer it to the centre of the prepared baking dish. Trim any excess from the bottom of the cauliflower to allow it to sit flat and upright.

Spread the onion, potatoes, and tomatoes in a single layer in the baking dish, surrounding the cauliflower. Brush the balsamic mixture all over cauliflower, saving some for basting. Use your hands to rub the glaze and remaining 1 teaspoon of nigella seeds into the cauliflower.

Roast the vegetables in the oven until they are tender, about 40 minutes, occasionally basting the cauliflower with the remaining glaze and turning the surrounding vegetables once, about halfway through. When the vegetables are tender, use a large spatula to carefully transfer them to a large serving plate. Garnish with parsley and serve hot.

ROASTED ROOT VEGETABLES ON GARLIC-BRAISED GREENS

MAKES: *4 servings*   DIFFICULTY: *Easy*

Garlicky dark greens are an ideal complement for the caramelized sweetness of the root vegetables.

ROOT VEGETABLES

1 parsnip, cut into 1-inch/2.5cm dice

1 carrot, cut into 1-inch/2.5cm dice

1 sweet potato, cut into 1-inch/2.5cm dice

1 waxy potato, cut into 1-inch/2.5cm dice

½ cup/75g chopped onion

½ teaspoon onion powder

¼ teaspoon ground black pepper

GARLICKY GREENS

⅓ cup/75ml Light Vegetable Broth (page 214) or water

3 to 4 garlic cloves, finely chopped

½ teaspoon dried oregano

¼ teaspoon red pepper flakes

2 teaspoons white miso paste

1 pound/450g dark leafy greens, tough stems removed, chopped

TO SERVE

Ground black pepper

FOR THE ROOT VEGETABLES: Preheat the oven to 220°C/425°F/gas mark 7. Line two roasting tins with silicone mats or baking parchment.

Evenly divide the vegetables between the prepared tins and spread them out in a single layer. Sprinkle with the onion powder and black pepper. Roast the vegetables in the oven until tender and slightly caramelized, 45 to 60 minutes, turning them with a metal spatula about halfway through. When the vegetables are done, remove the pans from the oven and set aside.

FOR THE GARLICKY GREENS: While the vegetables are roasting, combine the Light Vegetable Broth, garlic, oregano and red pepper flakes in a large pot and bring to the boil over medium-high heat. Lower the heat to medium and cook for 1 minute to soften the garlic. Stir in the miso paste, then add the greens and cook until wilted or tender. Depending on the type of greens, this can take as few as 3 minutes (for chard or spinach) or 25 to 45 minutes (for kale or collards). When the greens are tender, drain off any remaining liquid.

TO SERVE: Divide the greens among shallow bowls or serving plates. Top with the roasted root vegetables, sprinkle with black pepper to taste and serve hot.

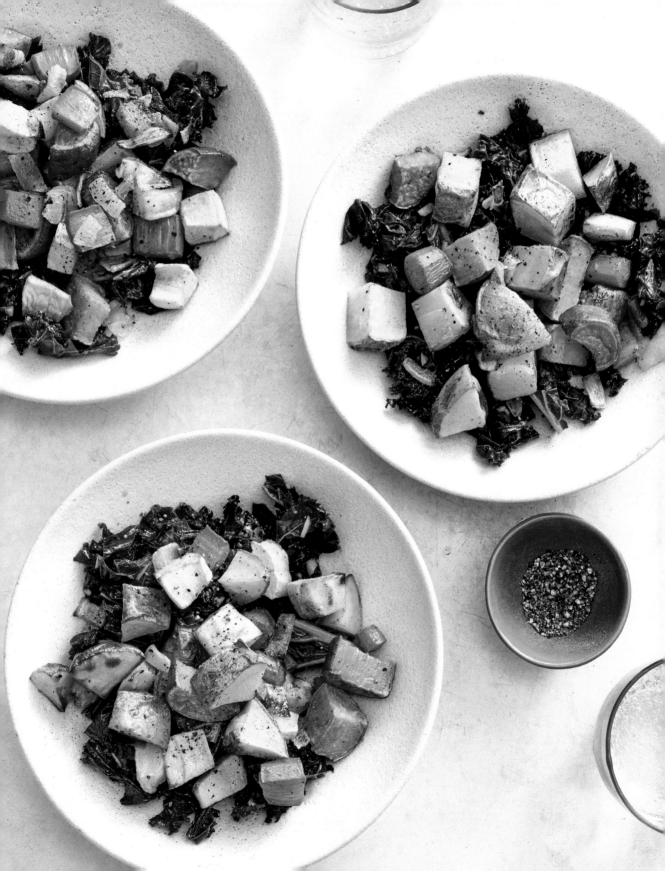

PORTOBELLOS AND SPINACH ON CAULIFLOWER MASH WITH MISO-MUSHROOM SAUCE

MAKES: *4 servings*   DIFFICULTY: *Moderate*

I like to make the mash and sauce ahead of time, so I can put dinner on the table in a flash.

CAULIFLOWER MASH

1 head cauliflower, trimmed and cut into 1-inch/2.5cm pieces

1 tablespoon nutritional yeast

1 teaspoon white miso paste

2 teaspoons Roasted Garlic (page 216) (optional)

SAUCE

2 shallots, finely chopped

2 cups/200g chopped assorted fresh mushrooms of your choice

2 tablespoons nutritional yeast

2 tablespoons white miso paste

1 teaspoon balsamic vinegar

1 teaspoon dried thyme

½ teaspoon dried sage

½ teaspoon onion powder

Ground black pepper

1½ cups/375ml Light Vegetable Broth (page 214)

MUSHROOMS

4 large portobello mushroom caps, stems and gills removed

3 spring onions, coarsely chopped

2 garlic cloves, finely chopped

1 teaspoon balsamic vinegar

½ teaspoon smoked paprika

Ground black pepper

6 cups/180g spinach leaves

TO SERVE

2 tablespoons chopped fresh parsley

FOR THE CAULIFLOWER MASH: Steam the cauliflower in a steamer basket over an inch or two (2.5–5cm) of boiling water until soft, about 10 minutes. Transfer to a bowl or a food processor and then add the nutritional yeast, miso paste and Roasted Garlic (if using). Mash or puree until smooth. Taste and adjust the seasonings, if needed. Keep warm.

FOR THE SAUCE: Heat ¼ cup/60ml of water in a saucepan over a medium heat. Add the shallots and cook until soft, about 3 minutes. Add the chopped mushrooms and cook for 2 to 3 minutes to soften. Add the nutritional yeast, miso paste, vinegar, thyme, sage, onion powder and black pepper to taste. Stir in the Light Vegetable Broth and bring to a simmer. Lower the heat to low and continue to simmer for 5 minutes. Transfer the mixture to a blender or a food processor and blend until smooth. Taste and adjust the seasonings, if needed. Return to the saucepan and keep warm.

FOR THE MUSHROOMS: Heat ¼ cup/60ml of water in a large skillet or heavy-based frying pan over a medium-high heat. Add the mushroom caps and cook for about 5 minutes. Add the spring onions, garlic, vinegar, smoked paprika and black pepper to taste. Flip the mushroom caps and continue to cook until the mushrooms are tender and nicely browned on both sides, about 5 minutes longer. When the portobellos are done cooking, push them to one side of the skillet, or remove them from the skillet, if you prefer. Add the spinach to the skillet and cook, tossing with tongs, until the greens are wilted. Return the mushrooms to the skillet to heat through, if needed.

TO SERVE: Spoon the cauliflower mash onto dinner plates. Top with the portobello caps, stem side down, and the spinach; then spoon over the sauce. Sprinkle with parsley and serve hot.

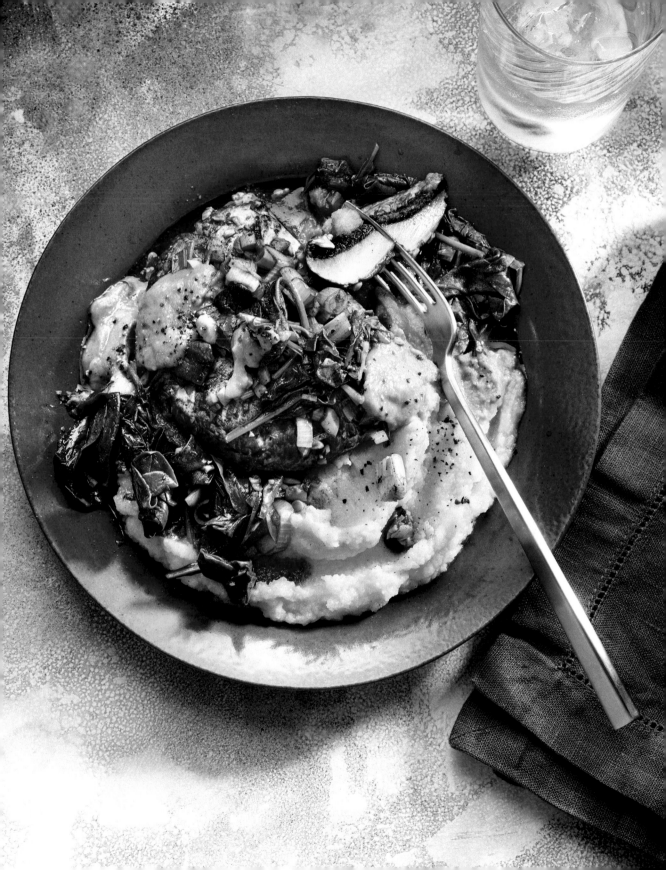

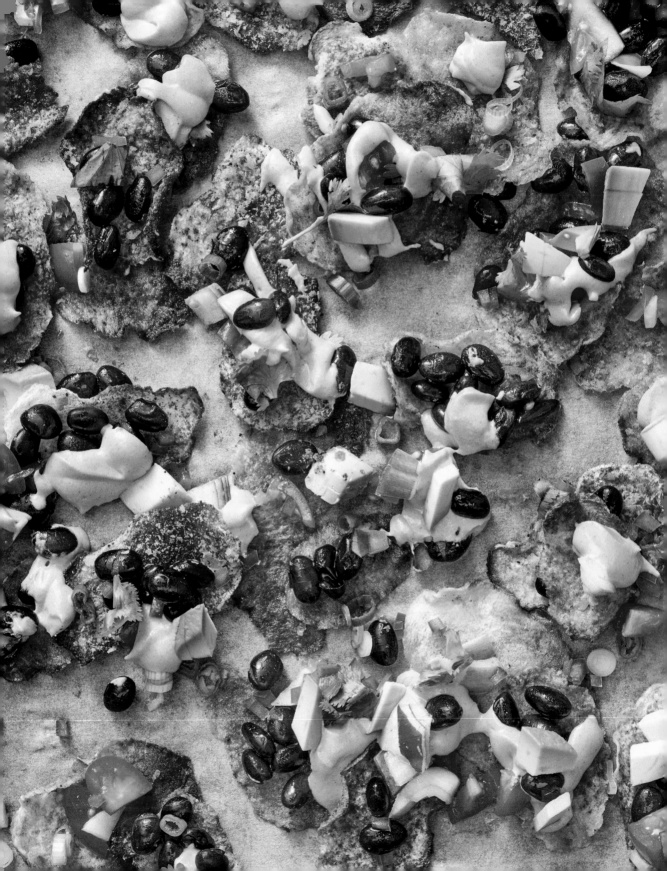

JICAMA NACHOS

MAKES: *4 servings*   DIFFICULTY: *Moderate*

Who doesn't love nachos? If you use jicama chips instead of greasy, salty tortilla chips, your heart will be as happy as your palate. Leftover queso sauce can be used to top cooked vegetable and whole-grain dishes, and it also freezes well, so consider doubling up when making that component – you'll have some on hand for another delicious meal. If you're not a fan of jicama, you can bake sliced potatoes instead. Alternatively, raw veggies, such as sliced peppers, carrots or cucumbers, can also be used to scoop up the tasty toppings.

JICAMA CHIPS

2 medium jicama, peeled

¼ cup/60ml fresh lime juice

1 tablespoon nutritional yeast

½ teaspoon onion powder

½ teaspoon garlic powder

½ teaspoon smoked paprika

QUESO

¾ cup/115g raw unsalted cashews, soaked for 30 minutes in hot water and then drained

Finely chopped jalapeño pepper, to taste

⅓ cup/45g nutritional yeast

1 tablespoon apple cider vinegar

2 teaspoons fresh lemon juice

1 teaspoon white miso paste

½ teaspoon smoked paprika

½ teaspoon onion powder

½ teaspoon garlic powder

½ teaspoon ground cumin

1 (¼-inch/5mm) piece fresh turmeric, grated, or ¼ teaspoon ground

NACHOS

1½ cups/250g cooked* or 1 (400g) BPA-free tin or Tetra Pak salt-free black beans, drained and rinsed

2 cups/500ml Fresh Tomato Salsa (page 210) or any salt-free salsa, drained

1 ripe Hass avocado, peeled, pitted and diced

3 tablespoons chopped spring onion

2 tablespoons finely chopped jalapeño peppers (optional)

⅓ cup/15g chopped fresh coriander

FOR THE JICAMA CHIPS: Preheat the oven to 200°C/400°F/gas mark 6. Line two large, rimmed baking trays with silicone mats or baking parchment.

Use a mandoline or sharp knife to slice the jicama into thin, crisp-size slices. Place the jicama slices in a bowl. Add the lime juice and toss gently to coat. Sprinkle with the nutritional yeast, onion powder, garlic powder and smoked paprika and toss gently to coat once again.

Arrange the seasoned jicama slices in a single layer on the prepared baking trays. Bake for 20 minutes, then remove the trays from the oven and turn over the jicama slices. Return the trays to the oven and bake for another 20 minutes, or until the edges are golden brown.

FOR THE QUESO: While the jicama slices are baking, combine all the queso ingredients plus ½ cup/120ml of water in a high-powered blender. Process until smooth, scraping down the sides as needed. Transfer to a saucepan and heat gently over a medium-low heat, stirring, for a minute or so. Taste and adjust the seasonings, if needed. Add a little more water if the queso is too thick. Keep warm.

FOR THE NACHOS: Warm the black beans on the stovetop or in a microwave until just hot. Set aside.

Evenly divide the jicama chips among four dinner plates and spread them out. Spoon about ⅓ cup/60g of black beans onto the centre of each plate and top with ½ cup/120ml of Fresh Tomato Salsa. Drizzle each serving with warm queso, as desired. Top with avocado, spring onion, jalapeños (if using) and coriander. Serve immediately.

*Turn to the Legumes and Grains Cooking Charts *on pages 218–221 for instruction, if needed.*

CAULIFLOWER PICCATA WITH MUSHROOMS AND POTATOES

MAKES: *4 servings*　　DIFFICULTY: *Easy*

These cauliflower steaks are simple to make, but you'd never know they didn't take hours and hours to create based on their complex flavours and gorgeous presentation.

---

1 head cauliflower, trimmed, cored, and cut vertically into ½-inch/1cm slices

8 ounces/225g small red potatoes, quartered

8 ounces/225g baby portobello mushrooms, trimmed and quartered

1 cup/150g cherry tomatoes

3 garlic cloves, crushed

2 teaspoons white miso paste

1 (¼-inch/5mm) piece fresh turmeric, grated, or ¼ teaspoon ground

½ cup/120ml Light Vegetable Broth (page 214)

3 tablespoons fresh lemon juice

3 tablespoons nutritional yeast

½ teaspoon onion powder

½ teaspoon salt-free stone-ground mustard

Ground black pepper

1 cup/175g cooked* cannellini beans, drained

4 spring onions, chopped

3 tablespoons chopped fresh parsley

Preheat the oven to 220°C/425°F/gas mark 7. Line a large roasting tin with a silicone mat or baking parchment.

Arrange the cauliflower slices and potatoes in the prepared roasting tin. Roast in the oven for 20 minutes, then remove the pan from the oven and turn over the vegetables with a metal spatula. Add the mushrooms and tomatoes, and return the tin to the oven. Roast until the vegetables are fork-tender and nicely browned, about 15 minutes longer.

Meanwhile, make the sauce. In a high-powered blender or food processor, combine the garlic, miso paste and turmeric and blend until the garlic is finely chopped. Add the Light Vegetable Broth, lemon juice, nutritional yeast, onion powder, mustard, black pepper to taste and white beans. Blend until very smooth.

Transfer the sauce to a small saucepan and heat over a low heat. Stir in the spring onion and parsley and taste to adjust the seasonings, if needed. Keep warm.

When the vegetables are done roasting, transfer them to a serving platter and spoon the sauce over the top. Serve hot.

*Turn to the Legumes and Grains Cooking Charts *on pages 218–221 for instruction, if needed.*

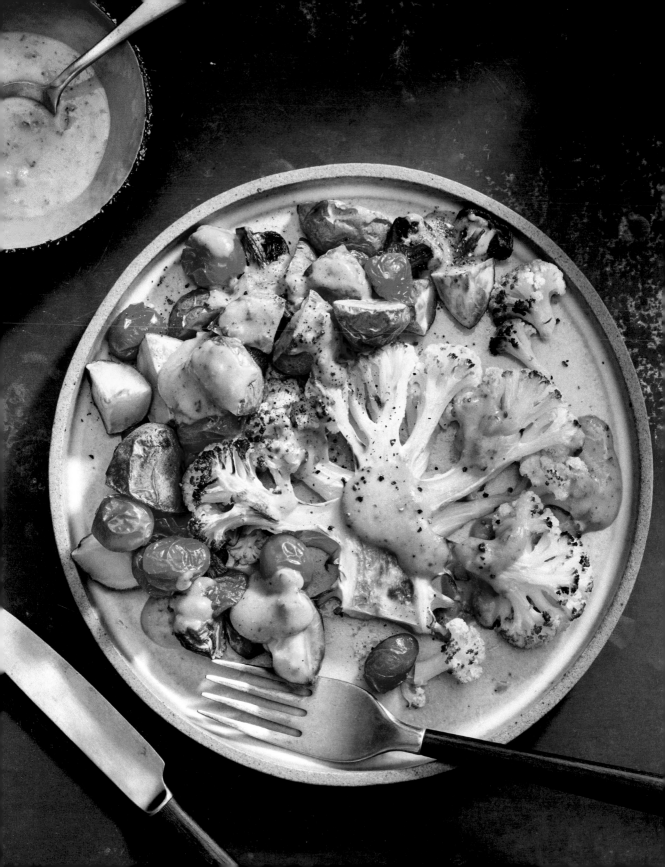

BALSAMIC BUTTERNUT, BRUSSELS AND BEETROOT

MAKES: *4 servings*   DIFFICULTY: *Easy*

If your beetroot comes with nice greens attached, consider cooking them up to serve as a bed for these beautiful alliterative veggies.

---

1 butternut squash, halved, de-seeded and cut into 1-inch/2.5cm dice (about 3½ cups)

1 pound/450g Brussels sprouts, trimmed and halved lengthways

1 bunch beetroot (3 to 4 medium beetroot, or about 1 pound/450g), trimmed and cut into 1-inch/2.5cm dice

1 red onion, cut into ½-inch/1cm dice

½ teaspoon dried oregano

½ teaspoon ground coriander

2 teaspoons Dr Greger's Special Spice Blend (page 212)

¼ cup/60ml Balsamic Syrup (page 215)

Ground black pepper

Preheat the oven to 220°C/425°F/gas mark 7. Line one or two large, rimmed baking trays with silicone mats or baking parchment.

Spread the squash, Brussels sprouts, beetroot and onion in a single layer on the prepared tray(s). Season with the oregano, coriander and 1 teaspoon of the Dr Greger's Special Spice Blend. Roast in the oven for 30 to 45 minutes, or until tender, turning the vegetables once, about halfway through.

Remove the tray(s) from the oven and transfer the vegetables to a serving dish. Drizzle with the Balsamic Syrup, season with the remaining 1 teaspoon of Dr Greger's Special Spice Blend and black pepper to taste and serve hot.

ARE GREENS AND BEETS BRAIN FOOD?

Our brain produces the artery-dilating compound nitric oxide, which is boosted by nitrate-rich vegetable consumption. After drinking 2 cups/500ml of beetroot juice, which has about as much nitrate as 2 cups/450g of cooked rocket, performance in a subtraction task was significantly improved, suggesting one dose of nitrate-rich vegetables can modify brain function. And our brain structure? Exercise alone may not result in any significant change, but, after the same amount of exercise and drinking some beetroot juice, there was a noticeable improvement.[56]

Can't *beet* that!

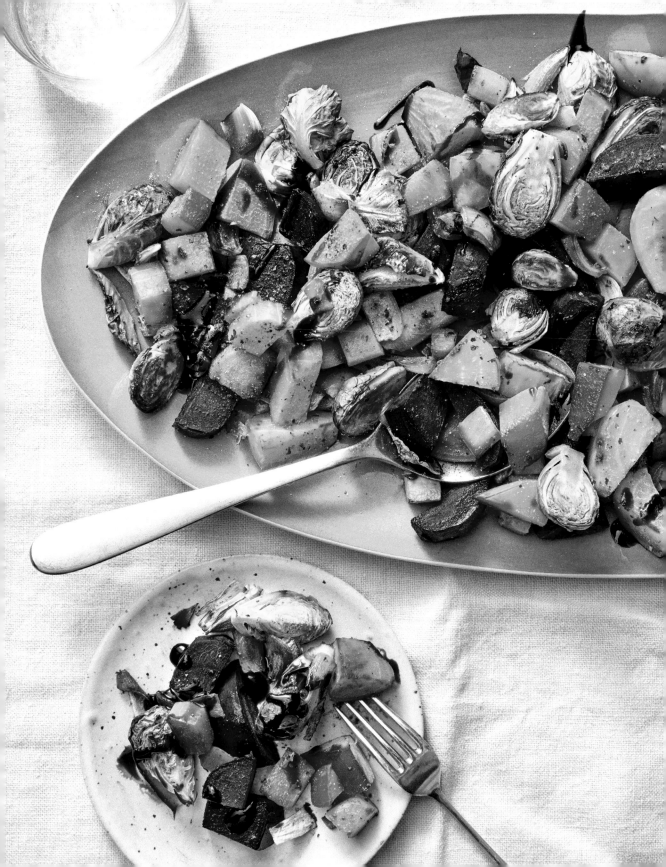

VEGETABLE TART

MAKES: *4 to 6 servings*   DIFFICULTY: *Moderate*

With two kinds of beans and loads of veggies, this beautiful tart with its chickpea crust has a lot going for it. Drizzle each serving with a little Balsamic Syrup to brighten the flavour even more. This will serve four as a main dish or six as a side dish.

CRUST

1½/250g cups cooked* or 1 (400g) BPA-free tin or Tetra Pak salt-free chickpeas, drained and rinsed, then blotted dry

2 tablespoons nutritional yeast

2 tablespoons ground chia seeds

1 tablespoon ground flaxseeds

1 tablespoon white miso paste

½ teaspoon garlic powder

½ teaspoon onion powder

1 teaspoon dried basil

½ teaspoon dried oregano

¼ teaspoon ground black pepper

FILLING

1 small red onion, finely chopped

1 small red pepper, de-seeded and chopped

3 garlic cloves, finely chopped

1 courgette, cut into thin rounds

6 ounces/150g white or baby portobello mushrooms, thinly sliced

4 spring onions, finely chopped

2 teaspoons white miso paste

1 teaspoon dried basil

1 teaspoon dried marjoram

¼ teaspoon ground black pepper

1½ cups/260g cooked* or 1 (400g) BPA-free tin or Tetra Pak salt-free white beans, drained and rinsed

3 tablespoons nutritional yeast

1 tablespoon apple cider vinegar

2 tablespoons ground chia seeds

½ teaspoon paprika

½ teaspoon onion powder

FOR THE CRUST: Preheat the oven to 200°C/400°F/gas mark 6. Cut a sheet of baking parchment to fit inside the bottom of a 9-inch/23cm springform tin. Line the tin and set aside.

In a food processor, combine all the crust ingredients and process until smooth. The mixture should hold together when pinched between two fingers. If it is too dry, blend in a little water, 1 tablespoon at a time. Transfer the chickpea mixture to the prepared tin. With damp fingers, press it down into the bottom of the prepared tin to spread it evenly. Bake for 10 minutes. Remove from the oven and set aside.

FOR THE FILLING: Heat ¼ cup/60ml of water in a large skillet or heavy-based frying pan over a medium-high heat. Add the onion, pepper and garlic and cook for 5 minutes to soften, adding a little more water if needed so the vegetables do not scorch. Stir in the courgette, mushrooms, spring onions, miso paste, basil, marjoram and black pepper. Cook, stirring, until all the vegetables are tender and the liquid has evaporated, 5 to 7 minutes. Stir to mix well; then remove from the heat and set aside.

In a blender or food processor, combine the white beans, nutritional yeast, apple cider vinegar, ground chia seeds, paprika, onion powder and turmeric. Process until smooth. Stir in the parsley.

Spread the white bean mixture evenly over the chickpea crust, and then spread the vegetables evenly over the top. Arrange the tomato halves, cut side down, on top of the vegetables in a concentric pattern around the edge, pressing the tomatoes

1 (½-inch/1cm) piece fresh turmeric, grated, or ½ teaspoon ground

2 tablespoons chopped fresh parsley

1 cup/150g cherry tomatoes, halved lengthways

¼ cup/25g ground walnuts (optional)

Balsamic Syrup (page 215)

into the vegetables. Sprinkle the top with walnuts (if using). Bake until hot and set, 18 to 20 minutes.

Remove from the oven and let the tart cool for about 10 minutes, then cut into wedges and serve hot, drizzled with Balsamic Syrup.

Turn to the Legumes and Grains Cooking Charts on pages 218–221 for instruction, if needed.

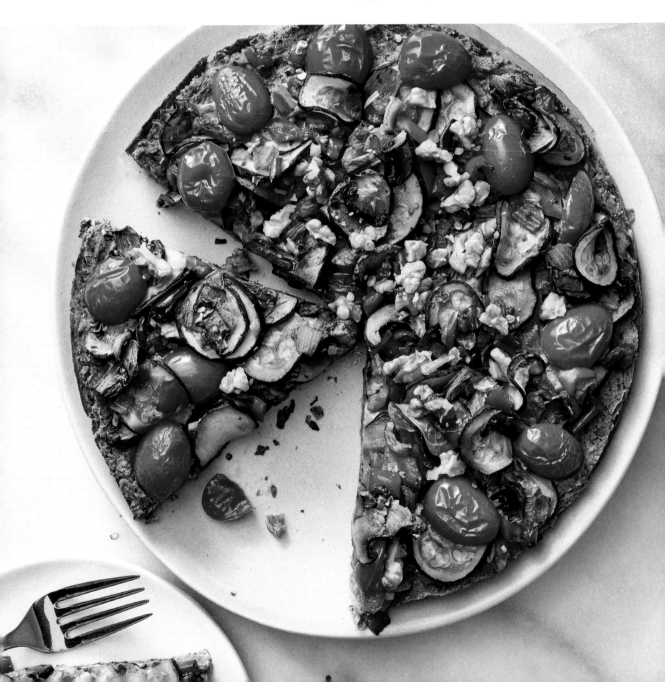

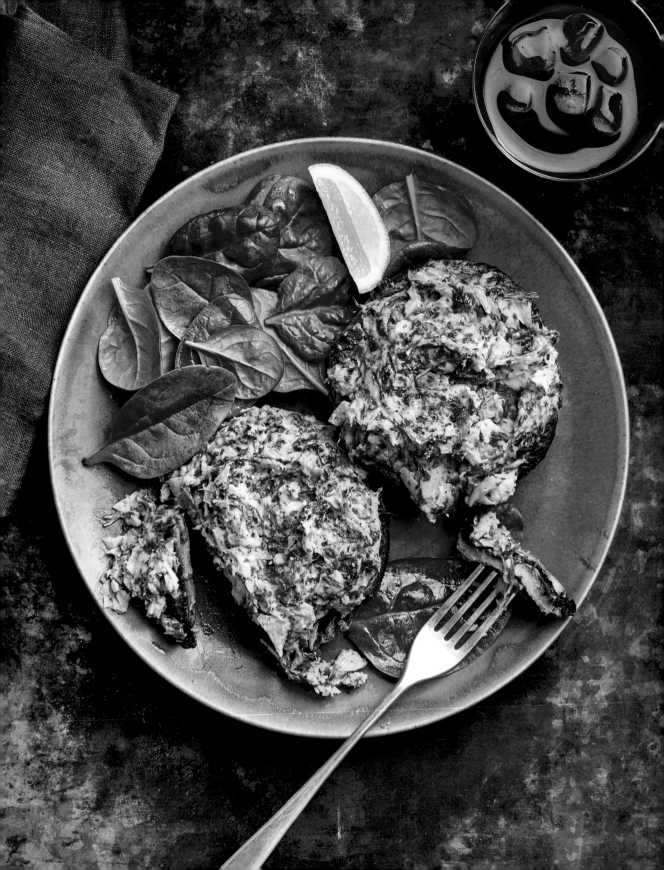

ARTICHOKE AND SPINACH STUFFED PORTOBELLOS

MAKES: *2 to 4 servings*   DIFFICULTY: *Easy*

If you like artichoke dip, a perennial favourite, you'll *love* this healthier and more flavour-packed version that we stuff into meaty portobellos. I like to serve two mushrooms per person as a main dish or one each as a side.

9–10 ounces/250–300g fresh or thawed frozen spinach, lightly steamed and cooled

1 cup/175g cooked* or BPA-free tinned or Tetra Pak salt-free white beans, drained and rinsed

2 tablespoons finely chopped spring onion

1 garlic clove, finely chopped

2 tablespoons nutritional yeast

1 tablespoon fresh lemon juice

1 teaspoon white miso paste

¼ teaspoon ground black pepper

1 (400g) BPA-free tin or Tetra Pak salt-free artichoke hearts, drained, or 1 (10-ounce/300g) package frozen artichokes, cooked and cooled

4 large portobello mushrooms, stems removed

2 tablespoons apple cider vinegar

½ teaspoon onion powder

¼ teaspoon ground black pepper

Squeeze the excess moisture from the cooled spinach and set the greens aside.

In a food processor, combine the white beans, spring onion and garlic and pulse until finely chopped. Add the nutritional yeast, lemon juice, miso paste and black pepper and process until smooth and well blended. Add the artichokes and pulse until they are chopped. Add the spinach and pulse to combine. Set aside.

Preheat the oven to 190°C/375°F/gas mark 5. Line a baking tray with a silicone mat or baking parchment.

Arrange the mushroom caps, stem side down, in the prepared tray. Whisk together the apple cider vinegar, onion powder and black pepper in a small bowl and brush it on the mushrooms. Bake for 10 minutes to slightly soften the portobellos. Remove the tray from the oven and set aside until the mushrooms are cool enough to handle. Gently flip the mushrooms and stuff them with the filling. Return the tray to the oven and bake the stuffed mushrooms for 15 minutes, or until hot throughout.

Remove the tray from the oven and serve the stuffed mushrooms immediately.

✳Turn to the Legumes and Grains Cooking Charts *on pages 218–221 for instruction, if needed.*

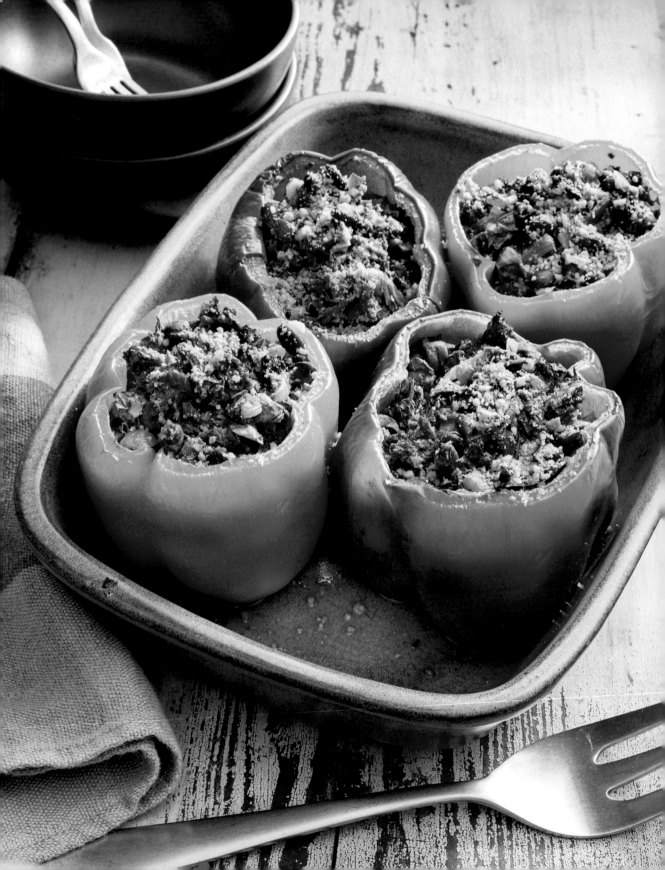

PEPPERS STUFFED WITH BLACK BEANS AND MUSHROOM–WALNUT CRUMBLES

MAKES: *4 servings*   DIFFICULTY: *Moderate*

The seasonings in this recipe give this stuffing a flavour similar to Italian sausage. Serve these stuffed peppers as is or top them with some warmed tomato sauce. (The Roasted Tomato Sauce on page 80 is my first choice, but your favourite salt-free marinara is fine.)

---

4 large peppers (any colour), tops cut off and seeds removed

1 small red onion, finely chopped

3 garlic cloves, finely chopped

4 cups/260g finely chopped kale

4 ounces/115g white mushrooms, chopped

1½ cups/250g cooked* or 1 (400g) BPA-free tin or Tetra Pak salt-free black beans, drained and rinsed

3 plum tomatoes, cored and finely chopped, or 1 (400g) BPA-free tin or Tetra Pak salt-free chopped tomatoes, drained and finely chopped

2 tablespoons nutritional yeast

1 teaspoon white miso paste

3 tablespoons finely chopped fresh parsley

½ teaspoon ground fennel seeds

¼ teaspoon red pepper flakes

¼ teaspoon ground black pepper

1 cup/120g Mushroom–Walnut Crumbles (page 208)

Warm tomato sauce (optional)

2 tablespoons Brazil Nut Parm (page 210)

Preheat the oven to 190°C/375°F/gas mark 5. Pour about 1 inch/2.5cm of water into a shallow baking dish and set aside.

Lightly steam the peppers on a rack set over boiling water in a large pot for 3 to 4 minutes, to soften them slightly. Remove the peppers from the steamer and set aside, cut side down, to drain.

Heat ¼ cup/60ml of water in a large skillet or heavy-based frying pan over a medium heat. Add the onion and cook until soft, about 5 minutes. Add the garlic and cook for 1 minute longer; then stir in the kale, mushrooms, beans, tomatoes, nutritional yeast, miso paste, parsley, fennel seeds, red pepper flakes and black pepper. Simmer over a medium heat for 10 to 15 minutes, or until the liquid is absorbed. Stir in the Mushroom–Walnut Crumbles and mix well to combine. Taste and adjust the seasonings, if needed. If the stuffing is too wet, add a little nutritional yeast or ground flaxseeds and combine well.

Fill the peppers with the stuffing, then place them upright in the prepared baking dish. Cover and bake until the peppers are tender, 25 to 30 minutes.

Serve hot, topped with the tomato sauce (if using) and sprinkled with Brazil Nut Parm.

Turn to the Legumes and Grains Cooking Charts *on pages 218–221 for instruction, if needed.*

ROASTED KABOCHA WITH KALE–CRANBERRY STUFFING

MAKES: *4 servings*   DIFFICULTY: *Moderate*

Rather than starchy, boring bread cubes, the stuffing for this dish is made with my Basic BROL (Barley, Rye, Oats and Lentils), combined with onion, celery, kale and cranberries. I like to serve it as is or topped with the Miso–Mushroom Sauce featured on page 102. To mix it up, try swapping in any combination of cooked whole grains with beans in place of the Basic BROL.

1 large kabocha squash, halved crossways (see Hint*)

½ cup/75g chopped red onion

½ cup/50g finely chopped celery

½ cup/50g cranberries

1 cup/30g finely shredded kale or other dark leafy greens of choice

1 tablespoon Umami Sauce Redux (page 212)

1 teaspoon finely chopped fresh thyme leaves, or ½ teaspoon dried

1 teaspoon finely chopped fresh rosemary leaves, or ½ teaspoon dried

1 teaspoon finely chopped fresh sage leaves, or ½ teaspoon dried

Ground black pepper

2 cups/360g Basic BROL (page 209)

Preheat the oven to 180°C/350°F/gas mark 4. Line a roasting tin with a silicone mat or baking parchment.

Using a strong knife, cut the cap off of the squash. With a spoon, scrape out and discard its seeds and fibres. Set aside.

Heat ¼ cup/60ml of water in a large skillet or heavy-based frying pan over a medium heat. Add the onion and celery and cook for 5 minutes. Stir in the cranberries, kale, Umami Sauce Redux, thyme, rosemary, sage and black pepper to taste. Remove from the heat and stir in the Basic BROL until well combined.

Spoon the stuffing into the centre of each half of the squash. Transfer the squash to the prepared roasting tin and bake for 1 hour 20 minutes. If the stuffing is getting too browned, cover it loosely with foil. Check the squash for tenderness after the baking time. If it cannot be pierced with the tip of a knife, return the the squash to the oven and bake for 15 to 20 minutes longer, or until the squash is soft and easily pierced with a knife. Serve hot.

Hint: To make a hard winter squash easier to cut, pierce the skin of the squash in a few places (to let the steam escape), then microwave it on High for 3 to 4 minutes. The squash will soften enough to cut easily.

BERRIES FOR INFLAMMATION AND OSTEOARTHRITIS

Higher intake of anthocyanins, berries' brightly coloured pigments, has been associated with anti-inflammatory effects, which may be a key component in reduced chronic disease risk.[57]

Can strawberries improve pain and inflammation in knee osteoarthritis? Yes! Simply adding berries to one's diet may have a significant impact on pain, inflammation, and overall quality of life.[58]

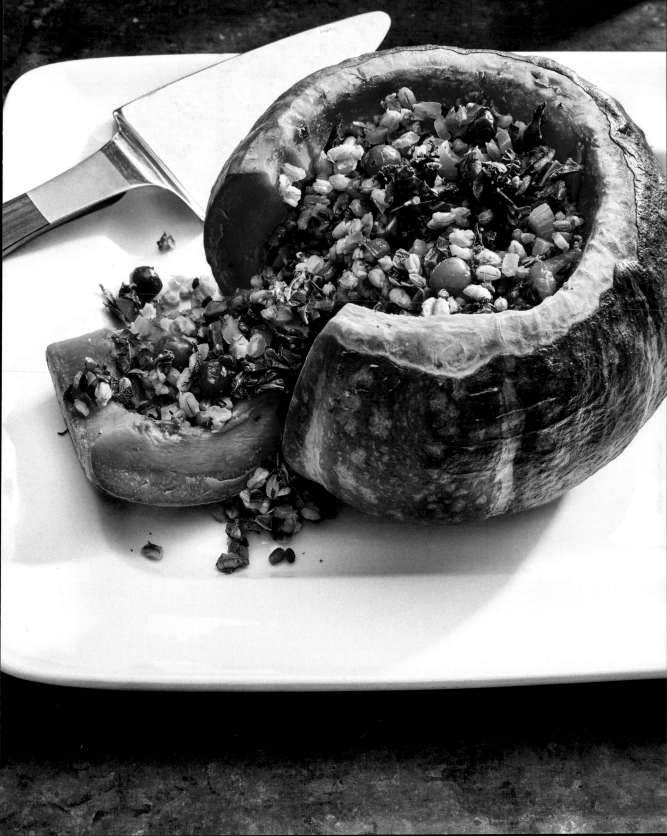

CUMIN-ROASTED CARROTS WITH CHICKPEAS AND TOMATOES

MAKES: *4 servings*   DIFFICULTY: *Easy*

Enjoy these savoury veggies as is, or serve over your favourite cooked whole grains or leafy greens. Roasting time depends on the size of your carrots – thinner carrots may be done in 20 to 25 minutes, while larger ones may take up to 45 minutes – so adjust accordingly.

1 pound/450g carrots, multicolour if available, cut diagonally into 1½-inch/4cm pieces

1½ cups/250g cooked* or 1 (400g) BPA-free tin or Tetra Pak salt-free chickpeas, drained and rinsed

Spritz of apple cider vinegar (see Hint**)

1 teaspoon ground cumin

1 teaspoon ground coriander

¼ teaspoon ground black pepper

3 cups/450g cherry tomatoes, halved lengthways

Cooked whole grains* or greens (optional)

¼ cup/4 tablespoons chopped fresh parsley or coriander

Preheat the oven to 200°C/400°F/gas mark 6. Line a large, rimmed baking tray with a silicone mat or baking parchment.

Spread the carrots and chickpeas in a single layer on the prepared tray. Spritz with apple cider vinegar and then sprinkle evenly with the cumin, coriander and black pepper. Roast in the oven for about 15 minutes, more or less, depending on the size of the carrots. Then, remove the tray from the oven and scatter the tomatoes over and around the carrots and chickpeas. Return the tray to the oven and continue to roast until the chickpeas are nearly crunchy and the carrots are tender and lightly charred, about 15 minutes more.

Serve in shallow bowls or plates over cooked whole grains or greens (if using), and sprinkle with the parsley. Serve hot.

*Turn to the Legumes and Grains Cooking Charts *on pages 218–221 for instruction, if needed.*

**Hint: *Keep a spray bottle handy with your favourite vinegar. Spritz vegetables before roasting to help spices adhere and to add a last-minute burst of flavour to salads and other dishes. I also give my air-popped popcorn a spritz or two so that nutritional yeast sticks on even better.*

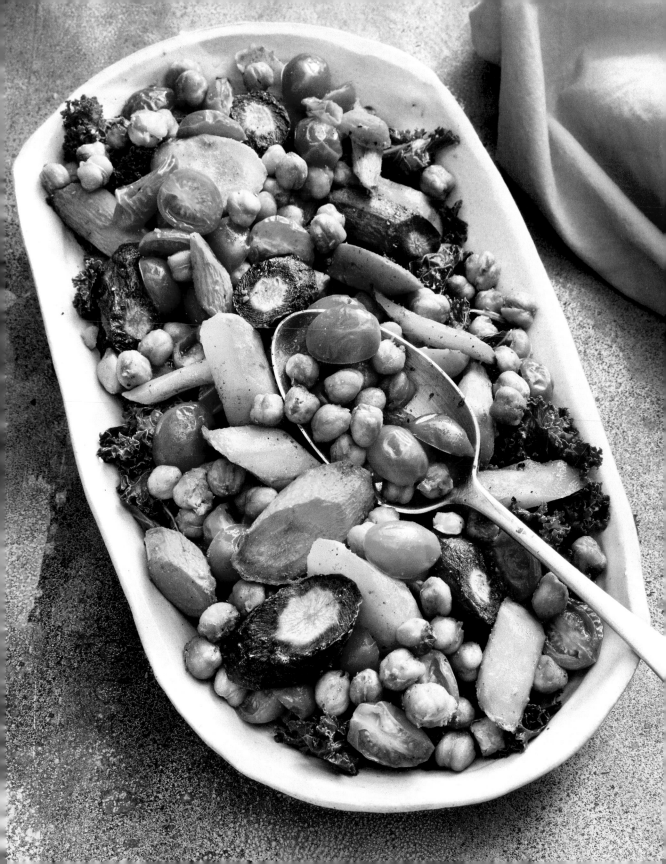

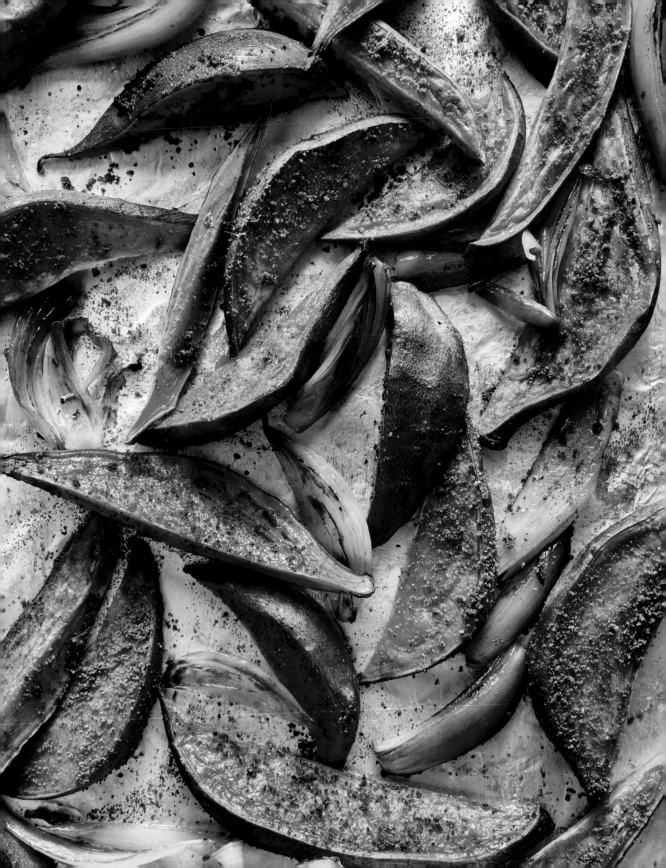

SAGE-KISSED SWEET POTATO WEDGES WITH SHALLOTS

MAKES: *4 servings*   DIFFICULTY: *Easy*

These roasted sweet potatoes are made even more flavoursome with the addition of malt vinegar, cornmeal and spices. If you prefer them unadorned, simply omit all the other ingredients and just roast the sweet potato wedges. They will still be delicious.

3 sweet potatoes (about 2 pounds/900g)

⅓ cup/50ml malt vinegar or apple cider vinegar, plus more to serve

⅓ cup/40g coarse cornmeal/polenta, blue if available

1 tablespoon smoked paprika

2 teaspoons ground sage

3 shallots, quartered lengthways (optional)

Preheat the oven to 220°C/425°F/gas mark 7. Line a large baking tray with a silicone mat or baking parchment.

Cut each sweet potato lengthways, into ½-inch/1cm wedges and place them in a bowl. Pour the vinegar onto the sweet potatoes and toss to coat.

In a small bowl, combine the cornmeal/polenta, paprika and sage. Mix well, and then sprinkle the seasoning mixture onto the sweet potatoes. Toss gently until evenly coated.

Arrange the sweet potato wedges in a single layer on the prepared tray, then distribute the shallots (if using) among them. Roast in the oven for 30 minutes, or until soft and lightly browned, turning over the sweet potatoes after 15 minutes. Serve immediately, with a little more vinegar if desired.

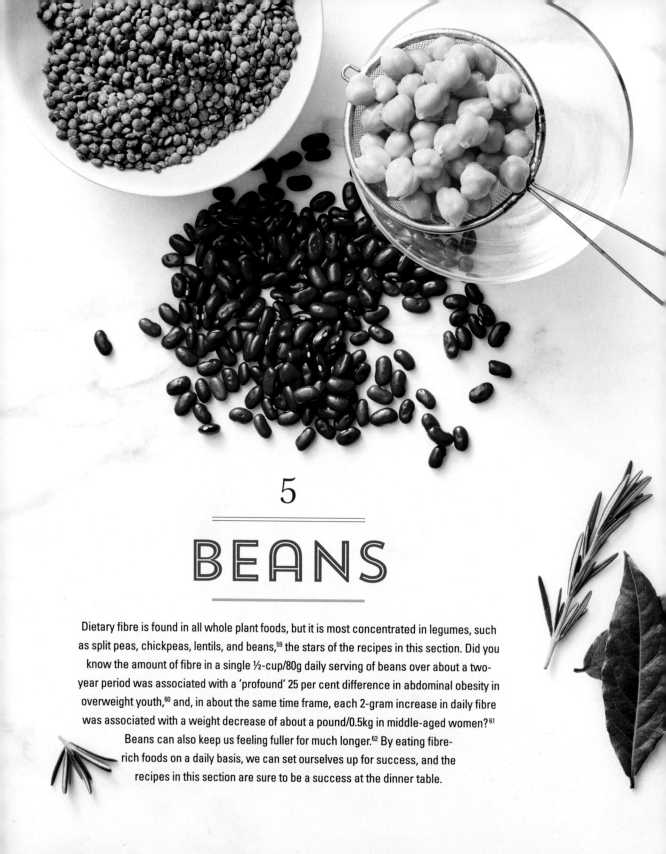

5

BEANS

Dietary fibre is found in all whole plant foods, but it is most concentrated in legumes, such as split peas, chickpeas, lentils, and beans,[59] the stars of the recipes in this section. Did you know the amount of fibre in a single ½-cup/80g daily serving of beans over about a two-year period was associated with a 'profound' 25 per cent difference in abdominal obesity in overweight youth,[60] and, in about the same time frame, each 2-gram increase in daily fibre was associated with a weight decrease of about a pound/0.5kg in middle-aged women?[61] Beans can also keep us feeling fuller for much longer.[62] By eating fibre-rich foods on a daily basis, we can set ourselves up for success, and the recipes in this section are sure to be a success at the dinner table.

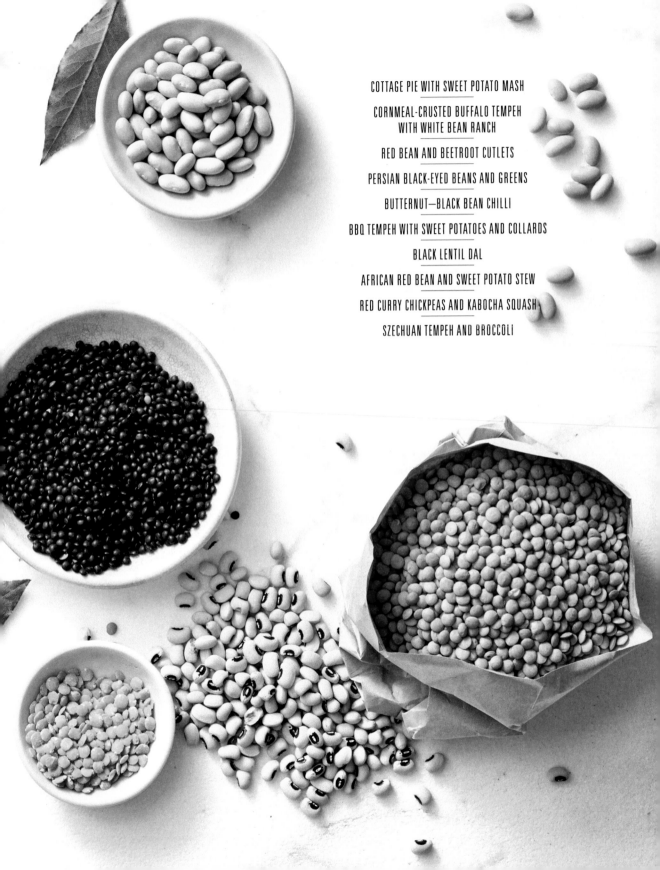

COTTAGE PIE WITH SWEET POTATO MASH

CORNMEAL-CRUSTED BUFFALO TEMPEH
WITH WHITE BEAN RANCH

RED BEAN AND BEETROOT CUTLETS

PERSIAN BLACK-EYED BEANS AND GREENS

BUTTERNUT—BLACK BEAN CHILLI

BBQ TEMPEH WITH SWEET POTATOES AND COLLARDS

BLACK LENTIL DAL

AFRICAN RED BEAN AND SWEET POTATO STEW

RED CURRY CHICKPEAS AND KABOCHA SQUASH

SZECHUAN TEMPEH AND BROCCOLI

COTTAGE PIE WITH SWEET POTATO MASH

MAKES: *4 to 6 servings*   DIFFICULTY: *Moderate*

One of my favourite comfort foods. This warm, savoury dish is just as flavoursome with mashed cauliflower instead of the sweet potato topping, so mix it up if the mood strikes.

2 pounds/900g sweet potato, cut into 2-inch/5cm chunks

½ teaspoon onion powder

¼ teaspoon ground black pepper

1 small red onion, chopped

1 carrot, chopped

2 garlic cloves, finely chopped

1½ cups/260g fresh or thawed frozen sweetcorn

1 cup/150g fresh or thawed frozen peas

1 cup/170g cooked* fresh or frozen broad beans

2 cups/400g cooked* or BPA-free tinned or Tetra Pak salt-free brown lentils

1 cup/250ml Light Vegetable Broth (page 214)

8 ounces/225g mushrooms of choice, chopped

3 tablespoons nutritional yeast

2 tablespoons salt-free tomato puree

1 tablespoon white miso paste

1 teaspoon finely chopped fresh thyme, or ½ teaspoon dried

Place the sweet potatoes into a large pot with enough cold water to cover and bring to the boil. Cook for 15 to 20 minutes, or until fork-tender, then drain and return to the pot. Stir in the onion powder and black pepper and mash until smooth. Set aside.

Preheat the oven to 200°C/400°F/gas mark 6.

Heat ¼ cup/60ml of water in a large skillet or heavy-based frying pan over a medium heat. Add the onion and carrot and cook until softened, about 7 minutes. Stir in the garlic and lower the heat to low. Stir in the sweetcorn, peas and cooked broad beans. Cook until the vegetables are tender and any liquid is absorbed, 3 to 5 minutes. Stir in three quarters of the lentils, then transfer the vegetable mixture to a shallow baking dish and set aside.

Heat the Light Vegetable Broth in the same large skillet over a medium heat. Add the mushrooms, nutritional yeast, tomato puree, miso paste and thyme and cook, stirring, for 5 minutes, or until the mushrooms are soft. Transfer the mushroom mixture to a blender or food processor, add the remaining lentils and blend until smooth. If the gravy is too thick, blend in up to ½ cup/120ml of additional broth. Taste and adjust the seasonings, if needed.

Pour the gravy over the vegetable mixture, stirring to combine. Spread the mashed sweet potatoes on top, smoothing to cover the surface. Bake for about 30 minutes, or until the filling is bubbling. Serve hot.

Turn to the Legumes and Grains Cooking Charts on pages 218–221 for instruction, if needed.

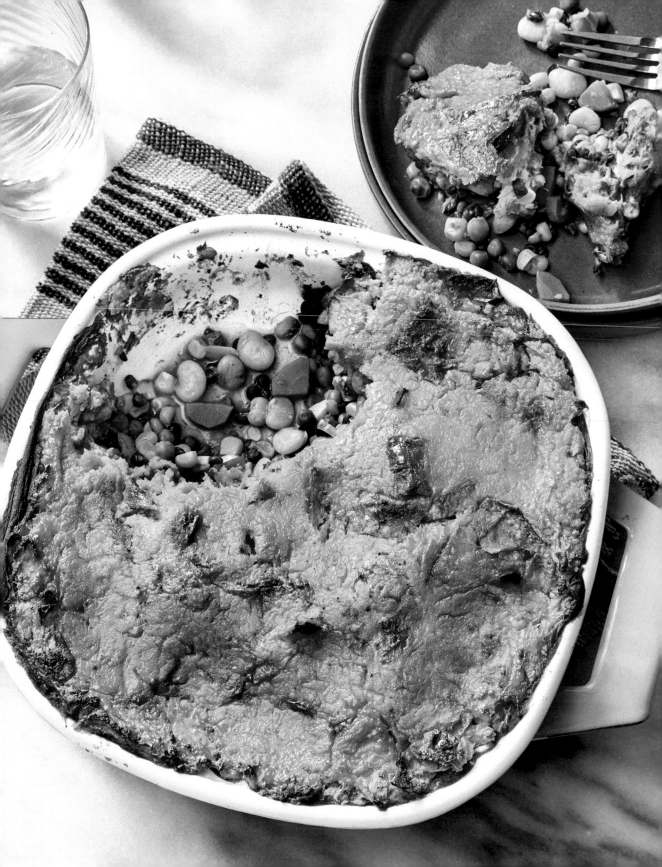

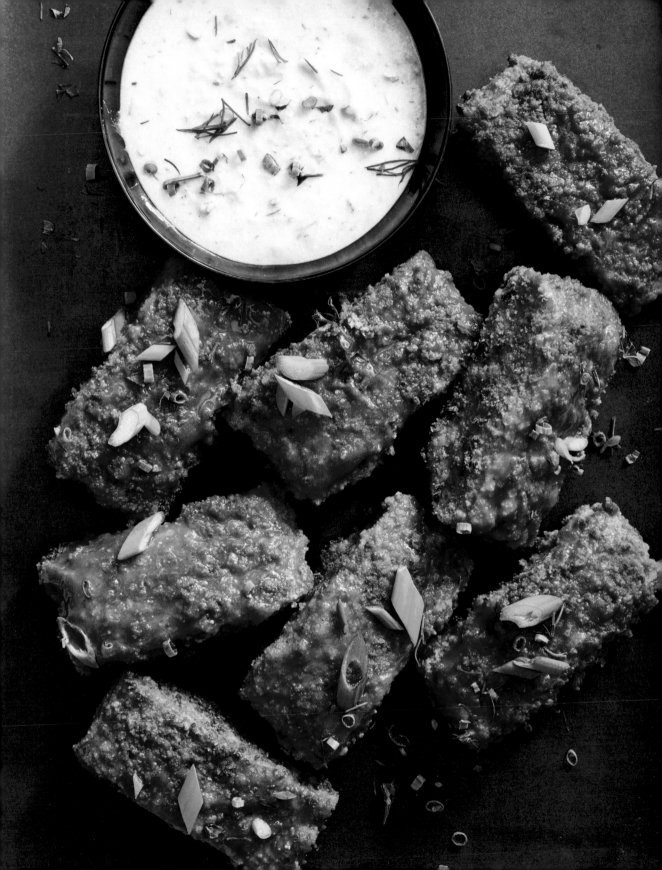

CORNMEAL-CRUSTED BUFFALO TEMPEH WITH WHITE BEAN RANCH

MAKES: *4 servings*   DIFFICULTY: *Moderate*

The White Bean Ranch isn't only the perfect dipping sauce for this tempeh dish – it also makes a great salad dressing.

WHITE BEAN RANCH

½ cup/90g cooked* or BPA-free tinned or Tetra Pak salt-free white beans, drained and rinsed

¼ cup/40g raw cashews, soaked for 30 minutes in hot water and then drained

1 tablespoon apple cider vinegar

2 teaspoons fresh lemon juice

1 teaspoon onion powder

½ teaspoon garlic powder

1 teaspoon white miso paste

¼ teaspoon ground black pepper

2 teaspoons finely chopped fresh parsley

1 teaspoon finely chopped fresh dill, or ¼ teaspoon dried

1 teaspoon finely chopped fresh chives, or ½ teaspoon dried

TEMPEH

¾ cup/90g coarse-ground cornmeal/polenta, blue if available

1 tablespoon nutritional yeast

1 teaspoon garlic powder

1 teaspoon Dr Greger's Special Spice Blend (page 212)

1 pound/450g tempeh, cut into 1- x 3-inch (2.5 x 7.5cm) bars

⅔ cup/150ml Salt-Free Hot Sauce (page 216), or more

FOR THE WHITE BEAN RANCH: In a high-powered blender, combine ⅓ cup/75ml of water with all the ingredients, except the parsley, dill and chives, and blend until smooth. Transfer the dressing to a bowl and stir in the parsley, dill and chives. Taste and adjust the seasonings, if needed, noting that the flavour will get stronger as the dressing sits. If the dressing is too thick, add a little more water and mix well. Cover and refrigerate for at least 1 hour to allow the flavours to develop. Stir or shake before serving.

FOR THE TEMPEH: Preheat the oven to 220°C/425°F/gas mark 7. Line a large, rimmed roasting tin with a silicone mat or baking parchment.

In a large bowl, combine the cornmeal/polenta, nutritional yeast, garlic powder and Dr Greger's Special Spice Blend. Stream in ¾ cup/175ml of water and whisk until smooth. Add the tempeh to the batter, turning to coat each piece. Arrange the battered tempeh pieces on the prepared tin but do not let them touch. Bake for 15 minutes, turning halfway through.

Pour the Salt-Free Hot Sauce into a large bowl. When the tempeh is done baking, remove it from the oven and gently toss it in the hot sauce to coat well. Return the tempeh pieces to the roasting tin and bake for 10 minutes longer, or until they become nicely browned.

Remove from the oven and let cool for 10 minutes before serving. If you like extra heat, toss the tempeh in additional hot sauce before serving.

TO SERVE: Place a small bowl containing the White Bean Ranch in the centre of a platter, surround with the tempeh, and serve.

Turn to the Legumes and Grains Cooking Charts *on pages 218–221 for instruction, if needed.*

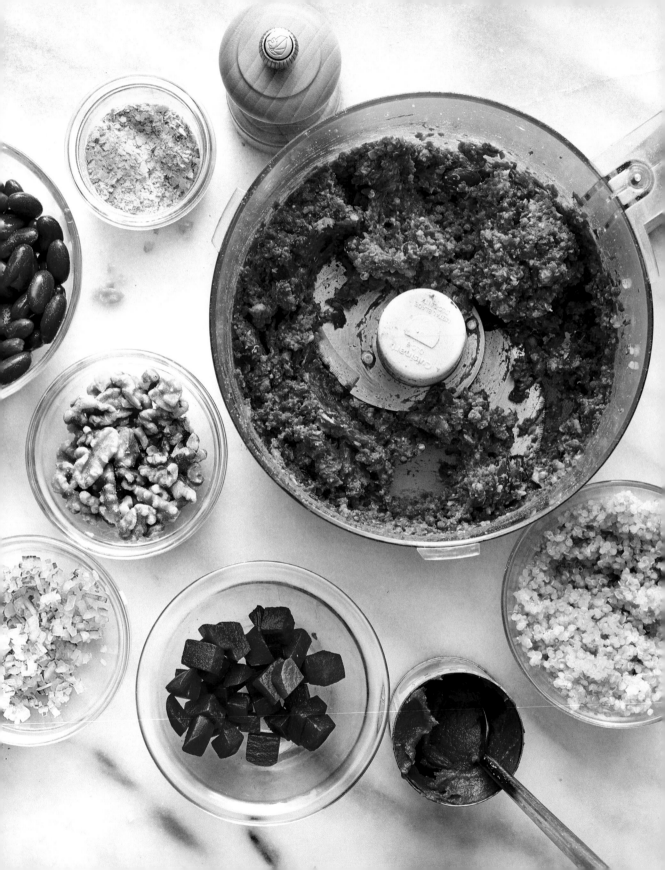

RED BEAN AND BEETROOT CUTLETS

MAKES: *6 servings*   DIFFICULTY: *Moderate*

Serve these cutlets on a bed of cooked greens. Enjoy as is, or top with your favourite sauce or a drizzle of Balsamic Syrup (page 215) or Umami Sauce Redux (page 212). These cutlets are also delicious served cold. Try slicing them and wrapping in lettuce leaves. This recipe is a great way to use up leftover cooked whole grains. If you don't want to roast or steam your own beetroot, look for precooked ones in the produce section of your supermarket.

1½ cups/260g cooked* or 1 (400g) BPA-free tin or Tetra Pak salt-free red kidney beans, drained and rinsed, then blotted dry

½ cup/60g chopped walnuts

¾ cup/140g cooked* quinoa, millet or other whole grain, blotted dry

½ cup/100g chopped roasted or steamed beetroot, blotted dry

¼ cup/40g finely chopped red onion

2 tablespoons nutritional yeast

2 tablespoons ground flaxseeds

2 tablespoons ground chia seeds

2 teaspoons salt-free tomato puree

¾ teaspoon Super-Charged Spice Blend (page 211), or to taste

½ teaspoon garlic powder

½ teaspoon onion powder

½ teaspoon smoked paprika

½ teaspoon white miso paste

¼ teaspoon ground black pepper

In a food processor, combine the beans, walnuts, cooked quinoa, beetroot and onion and process until well combined. Add all the remaining ingredients and process to mix well.

Transfer the mixture to a work surface and divide into six balls (or more or less, depending on how large you want your cutlets). The mixture will be soft. If it is too soft to handle, add a bit more ground walnuts or nutritional yeast and combine well. Use your hands to firmly shape each ball into a thin cutlet, pressing the mixture so the cutlets hold together. Set the cutlets aside on a plate and refrigerate for 1 hour or longer. (You may also wrap the cutlets tightly and freeze them for later use.)

Preheat the oven to 190°C/375°F/gas mark 5. Line a large baking tray with a silicone mat or baking parchment.

Arrange the cutlets on the prepared baking tray. Bake for 15 minutes, use a metal spatula to flip each cutlet; then bake for about 15 minutes longer, or until firm. Serve hot.

*Turn to the Legumes and Grains Cooking Charts on pages 218–221 for instruction, if needed.

PERSIAN BLACK-EYED BEANS AND GREENS

MAKES: *4 servings*   DIFFICULTY: *Easy*

A variety of fragrant spices turns a simple meal of beans and greens into something truly special. Black-eyed beans are available dried, frozen and tinned. If using dried or frozen, be sure to plan ahead to allow for enough time to cook them before you prepare the recipe.

1 large red onion, chopped

2 carrots, thinly sliced

2 tablespoons salt-free tomato puree

2 teaspoons white miso paste

1½ pounds/675g kale or collard greens, tough stems removed, coarsely chopped

2 cups/340g cooked* black-eyed beans

1 teaspoon ground coriander

1 teaspoon ground cumin

½ teaspoon dried fenugreek

½ teaspoon ground turmeric

½ teaspoon ground black pepper

½ teaspoon ground cardamom

¼ teaspoon ground cinnamon

⅛ teaspoon ground nutmeg or cloves

2 teaspoons fresh lemon juice

Hot cooked* whole grains (optional)

Heat ¼ cup/60ml of water in a large pot or deep skillet over a medium-high heat. Add the onion and carrots and cook until softened, about 5 minutes. Stir in the tomato puree and miso paste; then add the kale and 1 cup/250ml of water. Cover and simmer until the greens are tender, stirring occasionally.

Add the cooked black-eyed beans, coriander, cumin, fenugreek, turmeric, black pepper, cardamom, cinnamon and nutmeg. If the mixture is too thick, add a little more water to make it a bit saucy. Simmer for about 10 minutes to heat through and combine the flavours. Just before serving, stir in the lemon juice. Serve hot as is or over your favourite cooked whole grains.

Turn to the Legumes and Grains Cooking Charts *on pages 218–221 for instruction, if needed.*

HOW TO COOK GREENS

Although eating greens fresh is best, steaming's not bad, microwaving comes in second, and stir-frying and boiling fall to the bottom of the barrel.[63]

What about kale specifically? Blanching and steaming kale actually boost antioxidant content, whereas microwaving or even boiling doesn't seem to do much. So, you can boil kale without losing out on its antioxidant punch.[64]

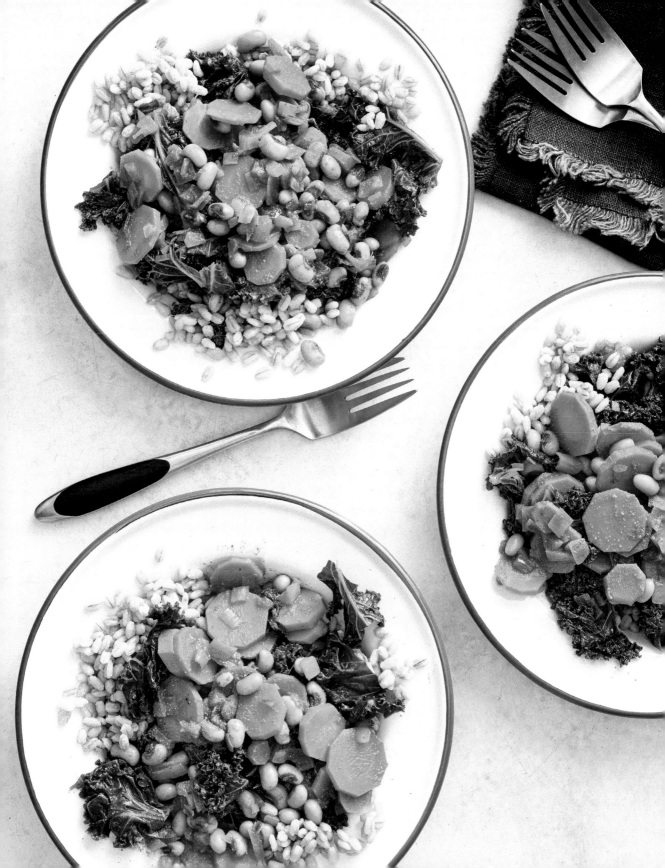

BUTTERNUT-BLACK BEAN CHILLI

MAKES: *4 to 6 servings*　　DIFFICULTY: *Easy*

Black beans marry chunks of butternut squash in this delicious chilli. If you won't have time to cut up a squash, look for diced squash in the produce section of your supermarket.

2 cups/500ml Light Vegetable Broth (page 214)

1 red onion, chopped

3 cups/420g peeled, de-seeded and diced butternut squash

1 pepper (any colour), de-seeded and chopped

2 garlic cloves, finely chopped

1 small hot chilli, de-seeded and finely chopped

¼ cup/4 tablespoons salt-free tomato puree

2 tablespoons chilli powder, or to taste

¼ teaspoon ground black pepper

1 (400g) BPA-free tin or Tetra Pak salt-free chopped tomatoes, undrained

3 cups/500g cooked* or 2 (400g) BPA-free tins or Tetra Paks salt-free black beans, drained and rinsed

2 tablespoons Umami Sauce Redux (page 212)

1 (¼-inch/5mm) piece fresh turmeric, grated, or ¼ teaspoon ground

1 tablespoon Super-Charged Spice Blend (page 211), or to taste

TO SERVE
Spring onions, chopped

In a large pot, heat 1 cup/250ml of the Light Vegetable Broth over a medium heat. Add the onion and cook until softened, stirring occasionally, about 5 minutes. Add the squash, pepper, garlic and chilli. Stir in the tomato puree, chilli powder and black pepper.

Add the tomatoes, black beans, Umami Sauce Redux, turmeric, Super-Charged Spice Blend and the remaining broth. Cover and simmer, stirring occasionally, until the squash is fork-tender and flavours have combined, about 45 minutes. Taste to adjust the seasonings, if needed, garnish with chopped spring onions, and serve hot.

＊*Turn to the* Legumes and Grains Cooking Charts *on pages 218–221 for instruction, if needed.*

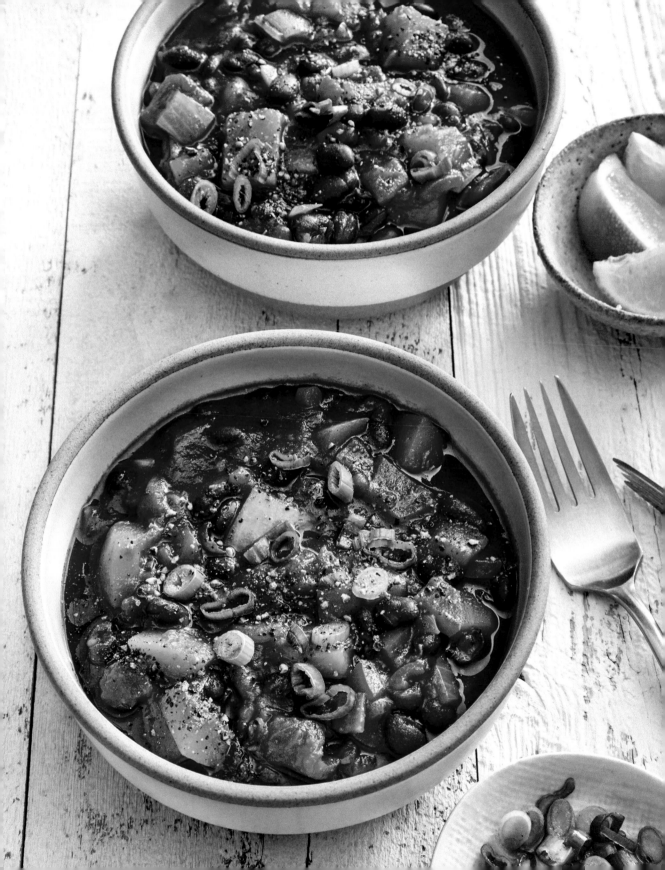

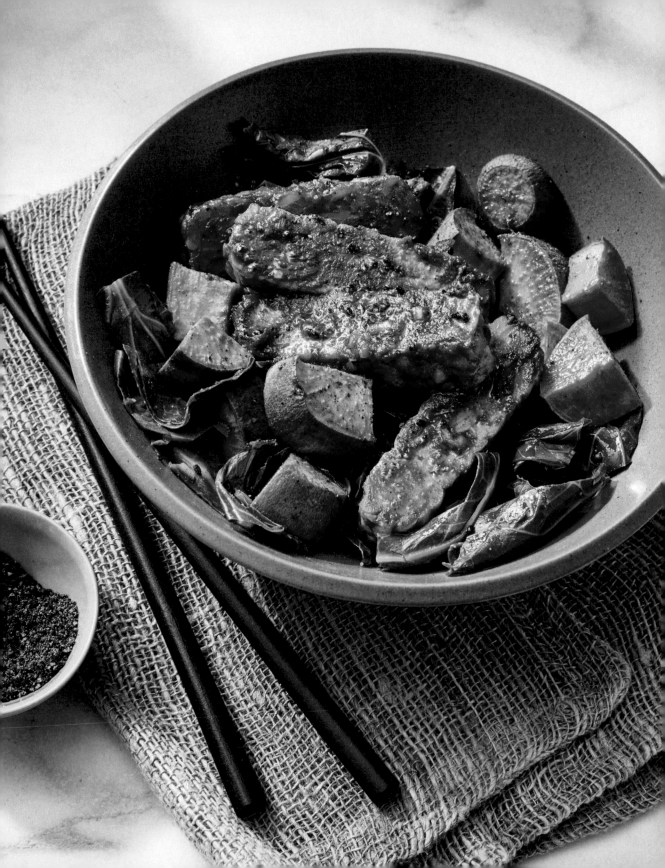

BBQ TEMPEH WITH SWEET POTATOES AND COLLARDS

MAKES: *4 servings*   DIFFICULTY: *Moderate*

This medley of collard greens, sweet potatoes and barbecued tempeh is a taste of the South served in one bowl. The dish is as delicious with kale in place of collards, so feel free to mix up your greens.

COLLARDS

1 small red onion, chopped

2 garlic cloves, finely chopped

1 teaspoon ground cumin

1 teaspoon smoked paprika

¼ teaspoon cayenne, or more to taste

Ground black pepper

2 cups/500ml Light Vegetable Broth (page 214)

1 bunch collard greens (about 12 ounces/350g), thick stems removed, coarsely chopped

Apple cider vinegar

SWEET POTATOES

2 large sweet potatoes, cut into 1-inch/2.5cm dice

Spritz of apple cider vinegar (see Hint*)

½ teaspoon onion powder

½ teaspoon smoked paprika

Ground black pepper

TEMPEH

8 ounces/225g tempeh, cut into ½-inch/1cm strips

1 cup/250ml Umami Sauce Redux (page 212)

2 tablespoons salt-free tomato puree

2 teaspoons salt-free mustard

TO SERVE

1 teaspoon coarsely ground nigella seeds

FOR THE COLLARDS: Heat ¼ cup/60ml of water in a large pot over a medium heat. Add the onion and cook for 5 minutes to soften. Add the garlic and cook, stirring, for 1 minute. Stir in the cumin, smoked paprika, cayenne and black pepper to taste. Add the Light Vegetable Broth and bring to the boil; then lower the heat to a simmer and add the collard greens, stirring to wilt. Cover and cook for 30 minutes. Uncover and continue to cook until the collards are tender and the liquid has mostly evaporated. When ready to serve, stir in a little apple cider vinegar. Keep warm.

FOR THE SWEET POTATOES: While the collards are cooking, preheat the oven to 220°C/425°F/gas mark 7. Line a large, rimmed baking tray with a silicone mat or baking parchment.

Arrange the diced sweet potato in a single layer on the prepared baking tray. Spritz the sweet potatoes with apple cider vinegar and season with onion powder, smoked paprika and black pepper to taste. Bake for 20 to 30 minutes, or until tender, turning once about halfway through. Keep warm.

FOR THE TEMPEH: Heat ⅓ cup/75ml of water in a large skillet or heavy-based frying pan over a medium heat. Add the tempeh and cook for 5 minutes, stirring occasionally. Stir in the Umami Sauce Redux, tomato puree, mustard and 3 more tablespoons of water. Lower the heat to low, cover, and cook for 15 minutes, periodically spooning the sauce over the tempeh to coat.

TO SERVE: Divide the collards among shallow bowls. Spoon the tempeh in the centre, and then arrange the sweet potatoes on either side. Sprinkle with nigella seeds and serve hot.

Hint: Keep a spray bottle handy with your favourite vinegar. Spritz vegetables before roasting to help spices adhere and to add a last-minute burst of flavour to salads and other dishes. I also give air-popped popcorn a spritz or two so that nutritional yeast sticks on even better.

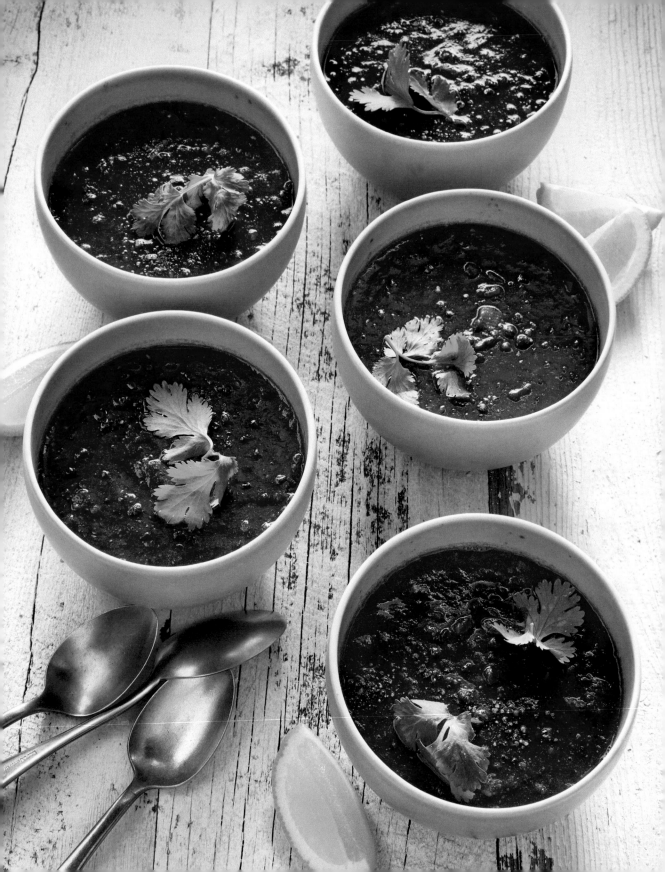

BLACK LENTIL DAL

MAKES: *4 servings* DIFFICULTY: *Easy*

Black lentils, also known as beluga lentils because they resemble caviar, stay perfectly intact when cooked and scatter well over salads. I like to serve this dal over my favourite cooked whole grains or greens. For variation, add one 400g BPA-free tin or Tetra Pak of salt-free red kidney beans to the dal for even more texture and colour.

1 red onion, finely chopped

3 garlic cloves, finely chopped

2 teaspoons grated fresh ginger

1 teaspoon garam masala

1 teaspoon ground coriander

½ teaspoon ground cumin

¼ to 1 teaspoon cayenne, to taste

1 (¼-inch/5mm) piece fresh turmeric, grated, or ¼ teaspoon ground

1 cup/260g salt-free tomato puree

2 tablespoons nutritional yeast

1 teaspoon white miso paste

1 cup/200g dried black lentils

4 cups/1 litre Light Vegetable Broth (page 214)

2 teaspoons fresh lemon juice

¼ cup/4 tablespoons chopped fresh coriander

Heat ¼ cup/60ml of water in a large saucepan over a medium heat. Add the onion and cook until softened, about 5 minutes. Stir in the garlic and ginger, cook for 1 minute, and then stir in the garam masala, coriander, cumin, cayenne to taste, turmeric and tomato puree. Cook for 2 minutes, stirring gently. Stir in the nutritional yeast, miso paste, lentils and Light Vegetable Broth. Bring to a simmer, then lower the heat to low, cover and cook, stirring occasionally, until the lentils are tender, 35 to 45 minutes.

For a creamier dal, blend half of the cooked dal in a blender until smooth, and then stir it back into the pot. Add a little water if the dal becomes too thick. Just before serving, stir in the lemon juice. Taste and adjust the seasonings, if needed. To serve, ladle into bowls and sprinkle the coriander on top. Serve hot.

THE BENEFITS OF LENTILS AND CHICKPEAS

Lentils and chickpeas have among the highest antioxidant content of legumes.[65] Lentils significantly slow stomach-emptying rates of meals eaten hours later,[66] and chickpeas may promote intestinal health,[67] so have some hummus with your lentil soup!

AFRICAN RED BEAN AND SWEET POTATO STEW

MAKES: *4 servings*   DIFFICULTY: *Easy*

Sweet potatoes and red kidney beans combine with a flavoursome peanutty broth for a healthier take on the classic African peanut stew. For a nice addition, stir in some cooked chopped greens near the end of the cooking time, long enough to heat through. Enjoy the stew as is, or serve over freshly cooked sorghum or another whole grain.

---

1 onion, chopped

1 red pepper, de-seeded and chopped

2 garlic cloves, finely chopped

2 teaspoons grated fresh ginger

½ teaspoon ground cumin

¼ teaspoon cayenne

1½ pounds/675g sweet potatoes, peeled and cut into ½-inch/1cm dice

1 (400g) BPA-free tin or Tetra Pak salt-free finely chopped tomatoes

2 teaspoons white miso paste

2 cups/500ml Light Vegetable Broth (page 214)

3 cups/525g cooked* or 2 (400g) BPA-free tins or Tetra Paks salt-free red kidney beans, drained and rinsed

2 tablespoons smooth unsalted natural peanut butter

¼ cup/30g chopped unsalted dry-roasted peanuts

½ teaspoon coarsely ground nigella seeds

Heat ¼ cup/60ml of water in a large saucepan over a medium heat. Add the onion, cover and cook until softened, about 5 minutes. Add the pepper and garlic, cover, and cook until softened, about 5 minutes. Stir in the ginger, cumin and cayenne and cook, stirring, for 30 seconds. Add the sweet potatoes and stir to coat. Stir in the tomatoes, miso paste and 1¾ cups/440ml of the Light Vegetable Broth. Bring to the boil, then lower the heat to low and simmer for about 20 minutes. Then, stir in the kidney beans and simmer until the vegetables are soft and heated through, about 10 minutes more.

Place the peanut butter in a small bowl and blend in the remaining ¼ cup/60ml of Light Vegetable Broth. Stir until smooth and then stir it into the stew. If a thicker consistency is desired, puree 1 cup/250ml of the stew in a blender or food processor and stir back into the pot. Taste and adjust the seasonings, if needed. Ladle into bowls, sprinkle with chopped peanuts and nigella seeds and serve hot.

Turn to the Legumes and Grains Cooking Charts on pages 218–221 for instruction, if needed.

ARE NON-STICK PANS MADE WITH TEFLON SAFE?

Non-stick pans seem like a great option since, well, food won't stick. But are they safe?

At normal cooking temperatures, Teflon-coated cookware releases various gases and chemicals that present mild to severe toxicity,[68]

and the coating itself can degrade over time, so some of the Teflon can chip off and make its way into the food.[69]

I'd stick with non-Teflon-coated pans to be safe.

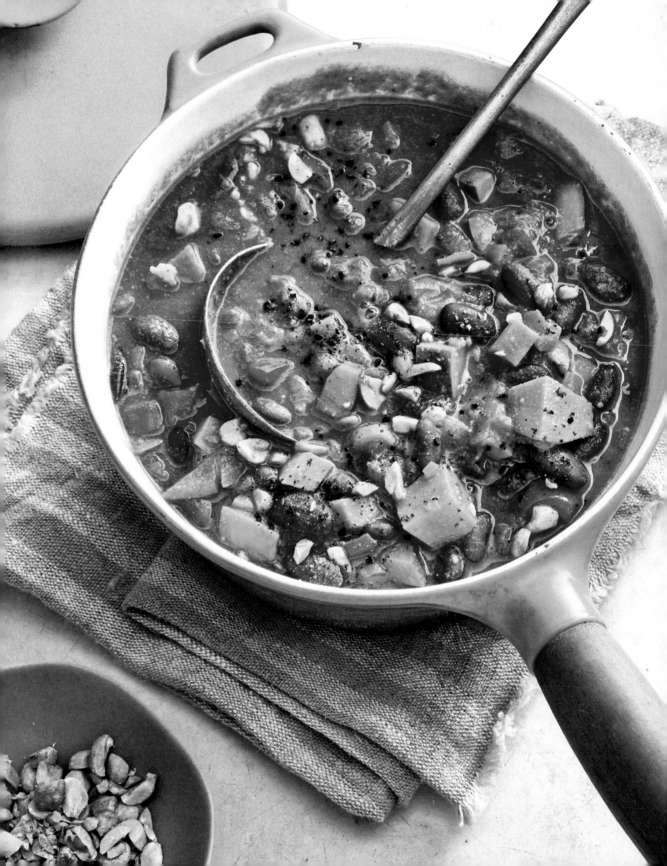

RED CURRY CHICKPEAS AND KABOCHA SQUASH

MAKES: *4 servings*   DIFFICULTY: *Moderate*

Turn this hearty dish into a robust meal by adding more veggies, such as cauliflower or green beans, to the curried chickpeas. Serve as is or on a bed of whole grains.

RED CURRY PASTE

2 red chillies, or more, to taste, de-stemmed and de-seeded

1 lemongrass stalk, tough parts removed, chopped

¼ cup/40g coarsely chopped shallot

1 tablespoon grated fresh ginger

3 garlic cloves, smashed

1 (1-inch/2.5cm) piece fresh turmeric, grated, or 1 teaspoon ground

3 tablespoons fresh lemon juice

SQUASH

1 large kabocha squash

1 teaspoon ground cumin

½ teaspoon ground coriander

CHICKPEAS

1 cup/250ml Light Vegetable Broth (page 214)

1 red onion, chopped

2 garlic cloves, finely chopped

1 green pepper, diced

1 (400g) BPA-free tin or Tetra Pak salt-free chopped tomatoes, undrained

2 tablespoons nutritional yeast

1 teaspoon smoked paprika

3 cups/500g cooked* or 2 (400g) BPA-free tins or Tetra Paks salt-free chickpeas, drained and rinsed

FOR THE RED CURRY PASTE: Combine all the curry paste ingredients in a food processor plus 2 tablespoons of water and blend to a paste. Taste and adjust the seasonings, if needed. Set aside.

FOR THE SQUASH: Preheat the oven to 200°C/400°F/gas mark 6. Line a large, rimmed baking tray with a silicone mat or baking parchment.

Place the whole squash on the prepared baking tray and roast in the oven for about 20 minutes. Remove from the oven and set aside until cool enough to handle.

Cut the cooled squash in half vertically, then use a spoon to scoop out the seeds and fibre. Cut the squash into eight uniform wedges. Arrange the wedges on the same baking tray and sprinkle with the cumin and coriander. Return the tray to the oven and bake for 20 minutes before removing the tray from the oven once again. Use a metal spatula to flip the wedges, and return the tray to the oven to bake the wedges until tender, another 15 to 20 minutes.

FOR THE CHICKPEAS: Heat the Light Vegetable Broth in a large pot over a medium heat. Add the onion and garlic, cover, and cook until tender, about 4 minutes. Stir in 2 to 3 tablespoons of the curry paste,** and then add the pepper and tomatoes. Cover and bring to the boil. Lower the heat to low and simmer until the vegetables are tender, about 20 minutes. When the vegetables are tender, use a hand blender to break up some of the vegetables or remove up to 2 cups/500ml of the solids and liquids from the pot, puree them in a blender or food processor, and return them to the pot. Stir in the nutritional yeast, smoked paprika and chickpeas and cook for 5 to 10 minutes longer to heat through and blend the flavours.

TO SERVE: Arrange the squash wedges on dinner plates or shallow bowls, two wedges per serving, and top with the curried chickpeas.

Turn to the Legumes and Grains Cooking Charts on pages 218–221 for instruction, if needed.

**Any leftover curry paste can be transferred to a jar or container with a tight-fitting lid and stored in the refrigerator or freezer.*

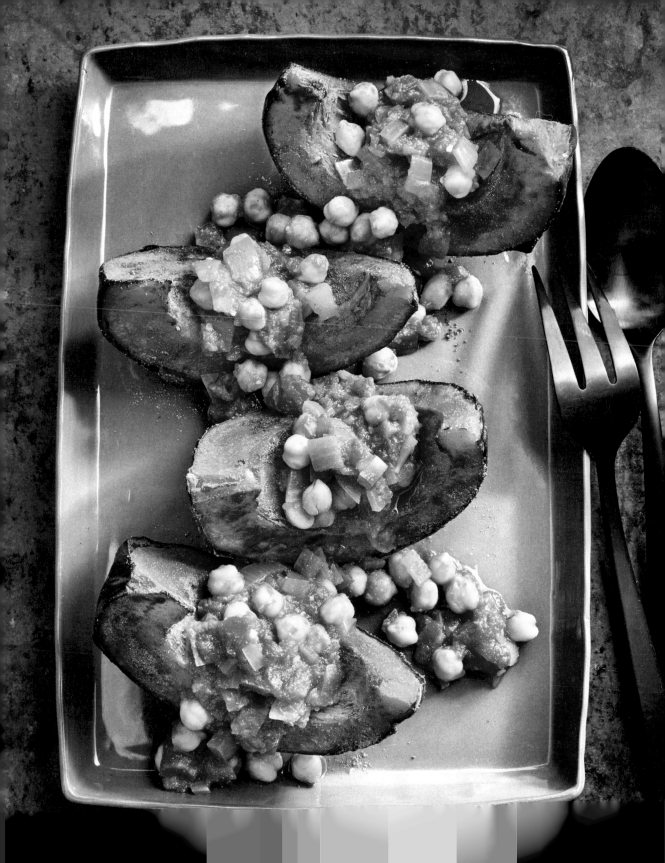

SZECHUAN TEMPEH AND BROCCOLI

MAKES: *4 servings*   DIFFICULTY: *Moderate*

Chinese takeout is often loaded with oil and sodium, but this version lets you enjoy classic Szechuan stir-fry at home without all of that grease and salt. Customize this recipe with a variety of your favourite veggies to suit your taste or to take advantage of what you have on hand.

MARINATED TEMPEH

8 ounces/225g tempeh, cut into ½-inch/1cm dice

2 tablespoons white miso paste

1 tablespoon apple cider vinegar

1 tablespoon Umami Sauce Redux (page 212)

½ teaspoon garlic powder

½ teaspoon ground ginger

¼ teaspoon cayenne

SZECHUAN SAUCE

¼ cup/60ml Umami Sauce Redux (page 212)

1 tablespoon treacle

2 teaspoons white miso paste

1 tablespoon rice vinegar

½ teaspoon Chinese five-spice powder

½ teaspoon garlic powder

½ teaspoon ground ginger

½ teaspoon red pepper flakes

STIR-FRY

1 head broccoli, cut into small florets

1 red onion, thinly sliced

1 red pepper, de-seeded, cut into strips

1 carrot, grated

3 garlic cloves, finely chopped

1½ cups/120g sliced mushrooms

2 spring onions, finely chopped

1 tablespoon grated fresh ginger

TO SERVE

Hot cooked* whole grains (optional)

FOR THE TEMPEH: Place the diced tempeh in a steamer basket over about an inch/2.5cm of boiling water and steam for 15 minutes. Set aside.

Pour all the remaining tempeh ingredients plus ¼ cup/60ml of water directly into a shallow bowl or freezer bag and mix well. Add the steamed tempeh and stir or turn the bag over a few times to coat the tempeh. Allow the tempeh to marinate at room temperature for about 45 minutes or in the refrigerator for 4 to 8 hours.

FOR THE SZECHUAN SAUCE: Combine all the sauce ingredients plus ⅓ cup/75ml of water in a small bowl or jar with a tight-fitting lid. Whisk or shake to blend well. Set aside. If not using right away, cover securely and refrigerate until you're ready to prepare the stir-fry.

FOR THE STIR-FRY: Heat a large, non-stick, Teflon-free wok or skillet over a medium-high heat. Add the marinated tempeh and stir-fry for 4 to 5 minutes, to brown all over. Remove the tempeh from the wok and set aside.

Place the broccoli florets in a steamer basket over about an inch/2.5cm of boiling water and steam lightly, 3 to 4 minutes. Set aside.

Add 2 tablespoons of water to the wok and reheat over a medium-high heat. Add the onion and stir-fry for 2 minutes. Add the pepper, carrot, garlic, mushrooms, spring onions and ginger and stir-fry for 1 to 2 minutes, or until softened. Return the browned marinated tempeh to the wok, add the steamed broccoli and stir-fry to combine. Stir or shake the Szechuan Sauce; then add it to the wok. Cook, stir-frying constantly, until the sauce coats the tempeh and vegetables, about 1 minute. Serve over freshly cooked whole grains of choice (if using).

*Turn to the Legumes and Grains Cooking Charts on pages 218–221 for instruction, if needed.

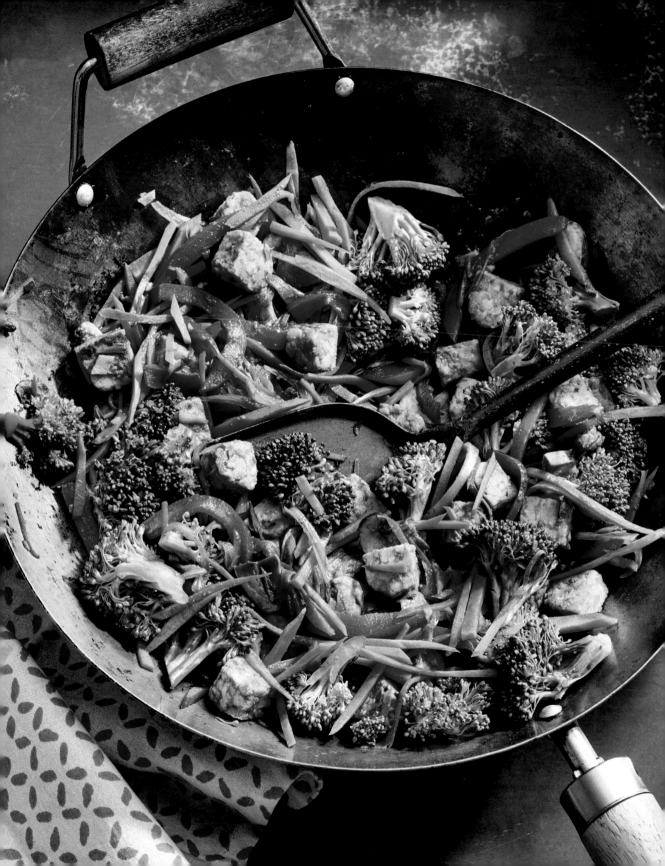

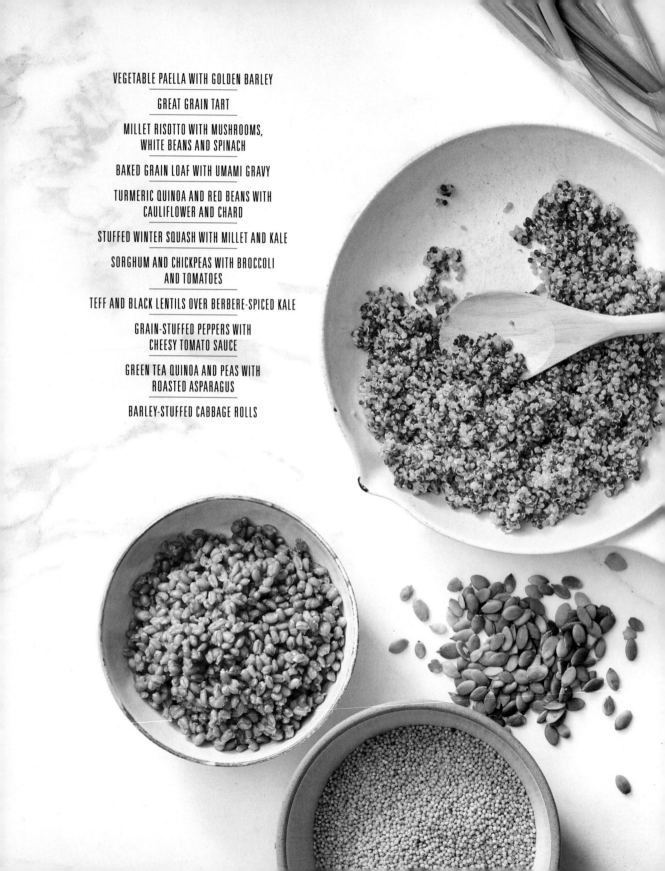

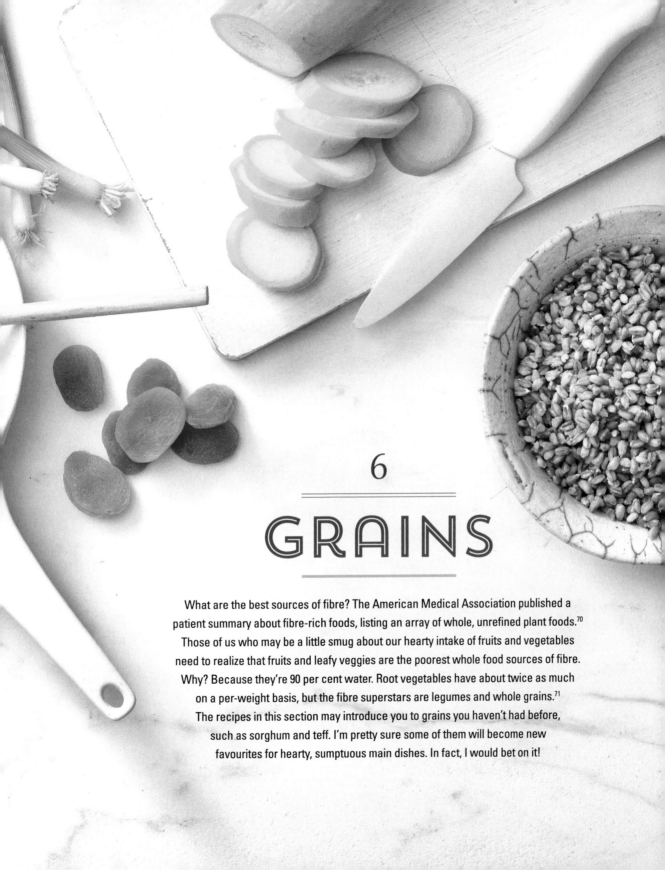

6

GRAINS

What are the best sources of fibre? The American Medical Association published a patient summary about fibre-rich foods, listing an array of whole, unrefined plant foods.[70] Those of us who may be a little smug about our hearty intake of fruits and vegetables need to realize that fruits and leafy veggies are the poorest whole food sources of fibre. Why? Because they're 90 per cent water. Root vegetables have about twice as much on a per-weight basis, but the fibre superstars are legumes and whole grains.[71] The recipes in this section may introduce you to grains you haven't had before, such as sorghum and teff. I'm pretty sure some of them will become new favourites for hearty, sumptuous main dishes. In fact, I would bet on it!

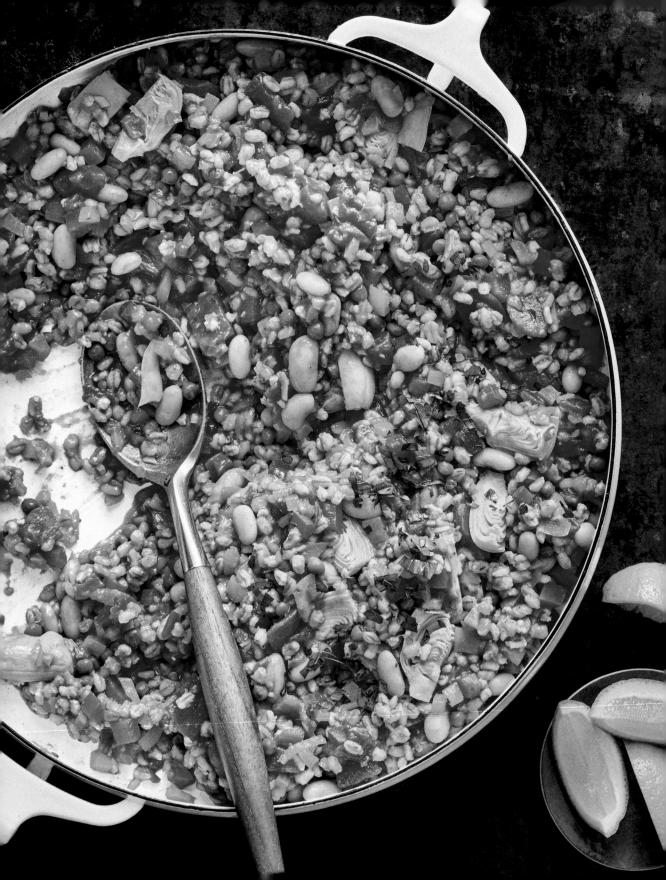

VEGETABLE PAELLA WITH GOLDEN BARLEY

MAKES: *4 to 6 servings*   DIFFICULTY: *Easy*

Paella is traditionally made with Spanish Valencia rice, but this version uses pot barley, which adds a chewy, nutty component to this flavoursome dish. Instead of the customary saffron, I use turmeric to achieve the same golden colour at a fraction of the cost.

3¼ cups/810ml Light Vegetable Broth (page 214)

1 onion, chopped

4 garlic cloves, finely chopped

1 red pepper, de-seeded and diced

1 yellow or green pepper, de-seeded and diced

2 (400g) BPA-free tins or Tetra Paks salt-free chopped tomatoes, undrained

1 cup/200g uncooked pot barley, soaked overnight in water and then drained

1 teaspoon smoked paprika

1 teaspoon ground fennel

1 (½-inch/1cm) piece fresh turmeric, grated, or ½ teaspoon ground

½ teaspoon dried oregano

¼ teaspoon red pepper flakes, or to taste

1½ cups/260g cooked* or 1 (400g) BPA-free tin or Tetra Pak salt-free cannellini beans, drained and rinsed

1 (400g) BPA-free tin artichoke hearts, drained and quartered

1 cup/150g peas

3 tablespoons chopped fresh flat-leaf parsley

1 lemon, cut into wedges

Heat ¼ cup/60ml of the Light Vegetable Broth in a large saucepan or paella pan over medium heat. Add the onion and garlic and cook until just softened, about 4 minutes. Stir in the red and yellow or green peppers, tomatoes with their juices, barley, paprika, fennel, turmeric, oregano and red pepper flakes. Stir in the remaining broth and bring to the boil. Lower the heat to a low simmer, cover, and cook until the barley is tender, 45 to 50 minutes.

Once the barley is tender, uncover, stir in the cannellini beans, artichoke hearts and peas, and then cover and set aside for 10 minutes before serving. Taste and adjust the seasonings, if needed. Sprinkle with the parsley, garnish with lemon wedges, and serve hot.

Turn to the Legumes and Grains Cooking Charts *on pages 218–221 for instruction, if needed.*

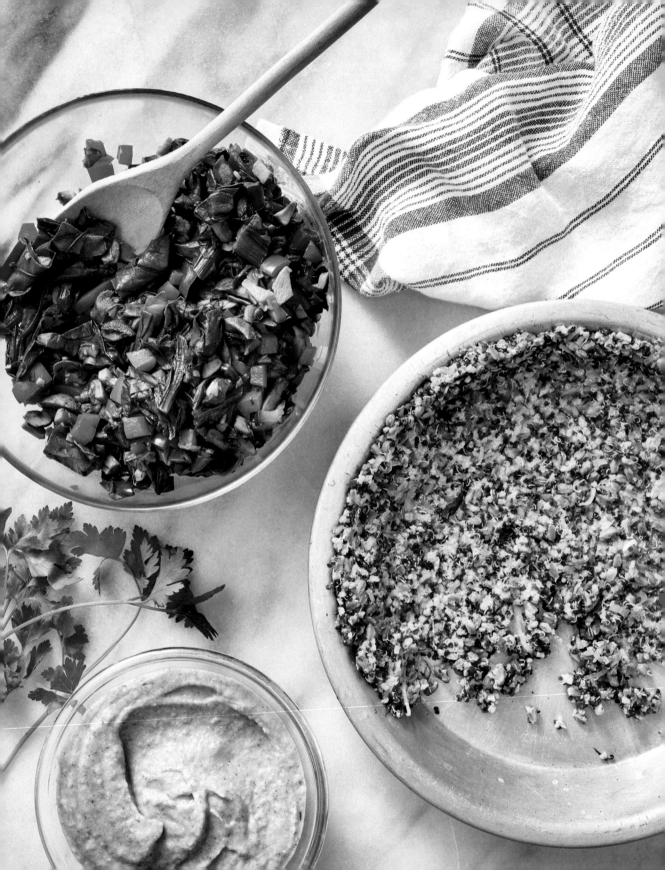

GREAT GRAIN TART

MAKES: *6 servings*   DIFFICULTY: *Moderate*

This tart is one of my go-to recipes when I want a delicious way to use up leftover cooked whole grains. Any combination works as well as the oat groats, quinoa and millet listed below, so feel free to be creative.

8 ounces/225g mushrooms, chopped

1 red or yellow pepper, de-seeded and chopped

3 garlic cloves, finely chopped

9 ounces/250g chard or spinach, chopped

2 tablespoons Umami Sauce Redux (page 212)

1 teaspoon smoked paprika

½ teaspoon dried thyme

Ground black pepper

½ cup/75g finely chopped red onion

1 celery stalk, finely chopped

3 tablespoons nutritional yeast

2 tablespoons ground flaxseeds

1 tablespoon white miso paste

1 teaspoon dried marjoram

1½ cups/260g cooked* or 1 (400g) BPA-free tin or Tetra Pak salt-free white beans, drained and rinsed

1 cup/160g cold cooked* oat groats

1 cup/185g cold cooked* quinoa

1 cup/175g cold cooked* millet

½ teaspoon onion powder

1 teaspoon garlic powder

3 spring onions, finely chopped

2 tablespoons finely chopped fresh parsley

2 tablespoons ground walnuts

1 lemon, cut into wedges (optional)

Heat ¼ cup/60ml of water in a large skillet or heavy-based frying pan over a medium-high heat. Add the mushrooms, pepper and garlic and cook until softened, stirring frequently, about 5 minutes. Stir in the chard, Umami Sauce Redux, paprika, thyme and black pepper to taste and cook for 3 minutes longer. Transfer to a bowl and set aside; then return the skillet to the heat.

Heat ¼ cup/60ml water in the same skillet and add the onion and celery. Cook over a medium heat until softened, about 5 minutes, stirring occasionally. Stir in the nutritional yeast, flaxseeds, miso paste and marjoram. Add the white beans and a little more water if needed, so the ingredients don't stick to the pan. Lower the heat to low and cook for 5 minutes, stirring occasionally. Remove from the heat and set aside to cool. Taste and adjust the seasonings, if needed. Transfer the mixture to a blender or food processor and blend until smooth.

Preheat the oven to 200°C/400°F/gas mark 6.

In a medium bowl, combine the cooked oat groats, quinoa and millet along with the onion powder, garlic powder, spring onions and parsley. Add about ¾ cup/175ml of the pureed white bean mixture and mix well. Evenly press the mixture into the bottom and up the sides of a deep-dish 9-inch/23cm pie plate to form the crust. Bake the crust for 10 minutes; then remove from the oven and set aside.

Add the remaining bean mixture to the chard mixture and mix well. Evenly spread the chard mixture over the crust. Sprinkle the top with ground walnuts and bake for 30 to 35 minutes, or until nicely browned.

Remove from the oven and let sit for at least 15 minutes before slicing. Serve warm or at room temperature with lemon wedges (if using).

Turn to the Legumes and Grains Cooking Charts *on pages 218–221 for instruction, if needed.*

MILLET RISOTTO WITH MUSHROOMS, WHITE BEANS AND SPINACH

MAKES: *4 servings*   DIFFICULTY: *Easy*

Millet isn't typically used to make risotto, but this recipe proves this healthy grain creates a delicious, creamy and savoury version.

3 cups/700ml Light Vegetable Broth (page 214)

½ cup/75g finely chopped red onion

2 garlic cloves, finely chopped

1 cup/200g uncooked millet

1 teaspoon white miso paste

2 cups/150g thinly sliced baby portobello mushrooms

1 cup/75g thinly sliced shiitake mushroom caps

1 tablespoon balsamic vinegar

¼ cup/35g nutritional yeast

1½ cups/260g cooked* or 1 (400g) BPA-free tin or Tetra Pak salt-free white beans, drained and rinsed

3 cups/75g chopped fresh spinach

Ground black pepper

Balsamic Syrup (page 215)

Heat ¼ cup/60ml of the Light Vegetable Broth in a large saucepan or deep skillet over a medium heat. Add the onion and cook for 5 minutes. Add the garlic and cook until fragrant, about 1 minute. Stir in the millet, miso paste, and the remaining broth. Bring just to the boil, then lower the heat to low, cover, and simmer for 30 minutes, or until the broth is absorbed and the millet is tender.

Meanwhile, heat 2 tablespoons of water in a large skillet or heavy-based frying pan over a medium-high heat. Add the baby portobello and shiitake mushrooms and cook, stirring occasionally, until lightly browned and softened, about 5 minutes. Add the vinegar and toss gently to coat the mushrooms. Remove the skillet from the heat and set aside.

When the millet is cooked, remove from the heat. Add the mushrooms and stir in the nutritional yeast, white beans and spinach, cover, and let stand for another 10 minutes.

Uncover and fluff the millet risotto with a fork. Spoon into shallow bowls, sprinkle with black pepper to taste, and serve hot, drizzled with Balsamic Syrup.

Turn to the Legumes and Grains Cooking Charts *on pages 218–221 for instruction, if needed.*

WHAT ABOUT MILLET?

Millet is a generic term applicable to many small grains,[72] such as pearl millet, which most of us think of as millet. But there are also proso, foxtail and finger millets, plus dozens of others. Much of its starch may be resistant starch that feeds the good bugs in our colon.[73] Millet also tends to have markedly slower stomach-emptying times than other starchy foods such as white rice, boiled potatoes or pasta.[74]

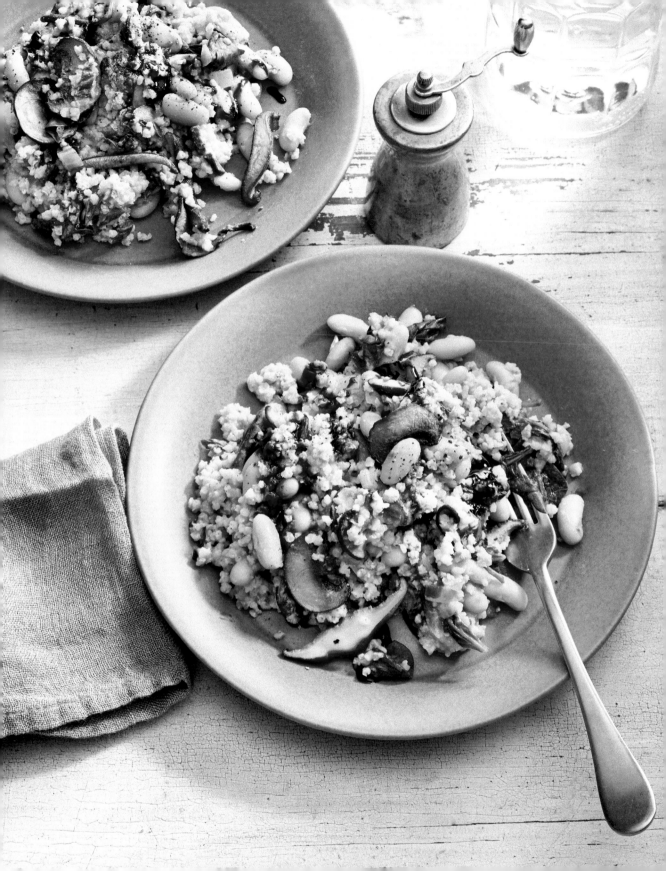

BAKED GRAIN LOAF WITH UMAMI GRAVY

MAKES: *6 servings*   DIFFICULTY: *Moderate*

This hearty loaf calls for small amounts of different cooked whole grains. I like to mix up the variety from time to time to use up leftovers or take advantage of what I have in my pantry. If I'm in a hurry and don't have leftovers or a lot of time to cook, I just substitute cooked Basic BROL (page 209) for the grains and lentils, since that's a staple I nearly always have on hand. Because the oven will be used for this dish, consider roasting some veggies to serve on the side.

LOAF

½ cup/75g chopped red onion

1 garlic clove, smashed

½ cup/60g walnut pieces

2 cups/320g cooked* barley groats or oat groats

1 cup/185g cooked* red quinoa

1½ cups/300g cooked* brown lentils

2 tablespoons tahini

3 tablespoons nutritional yeast

2 tablespoons ground flaxseeds

1 tablespoon finely chopped fresh parsley

1 tablespoon white miso paste

1 teaspoon smoked paprika

½ teaspoon dried thyme

½ teaspoon dried sage

¼ teaspoon ground black pepper

UMAMI GRAVY

1 cup/250ml Light Vegetable Broth (page 214)

2 shallots, finely chopped

2 garlic cloves, finely chopped

1 cup /100g chopped baby portobello mushrooms

2 tablespoons Umami Sauce Redux (page 212)

2 tablespoons nutritional yeast

1 tablespoon white miso paste

1 tablespoon salt-free tomato puree

1 teaspoon balsamic vinegar

FOR THE LOAF: Preheat the oven to 180°C/350°F/gas mark 4. Line an 8- x 4-inch/10 x 20cm loaf tin with a piece of baking parchment the same length of the tin and long enough to come over the sides by a few inches/5cm.

Combine the onion, garlic and walnuts in a food processor and pulse until finely chopped. Add all the remaining loaf ingredients and process until well combined. If the mixture is too wet to hold together, add more nutritional yeast or ground walnuts and combine well.

Transfer the loaf mixture into the prepared tin. Press the mixture firmly into the tin and smooth out the top. Bake until firm and golden brown, 50 to 60 minutes. Check its progress at around 40 minutes and if the top is getting too brown, cover with foil for the remaining baking time.

FOR THE UMAMI GRAVY: While the loaf is baking, make the gravy. In a saucepan, combine the Light Vegetable Broth, shallots, garlic and mushrooms and bring to the boil. Lower the heat to a simmer, stir in the remaining ingredients, cover, and simmer for 5 minutes. Transfer the mixture to a blender or food processor and blend until smooth. Return the gravy to the saucepan and taste and adjust the seasonings, if needed.

IS ALUMINIUM SAFE?

Consumers using aluminium cookware had twice the level of aluminium in their blood, and those with the highest levels tended to suffer significantly more damage to their DNA.[75] Occasionally using aluminium pots, utensils, and bottles may not be problematic, but regular daily use isn't ideal.

And foil? Foil leaks into food, but it's more of an issue for young children or those suffering from diminished kidney function.[76]

1 teaspoon dried thyme

½ teaspoon onion powder

½ teaspoon dried sage

¼ teaspoon ground black pepper

1½ cups/250g cooked* or 1 (400g) BPA-free tin or Tetra Pak salt-free black beans, drained and rinsed

Keep warm over low heat, stirring occasionally.

TO SERVE: When the loaf is done, remove from the oven, uncover if necessary, and let stand for 10 minutes before slicing. Run a knife down the long sides of the tin to loosen the loaf. Grasp the end flaps of the baking parchment to help lift the loaf out of the tin. Slice the loaf with a long serrated knife, top each slice with the gravy, and serve hot.

*Turn to the Legumes and Grains Cooking Charts *on pages 218–221 for instruction, if needed.*

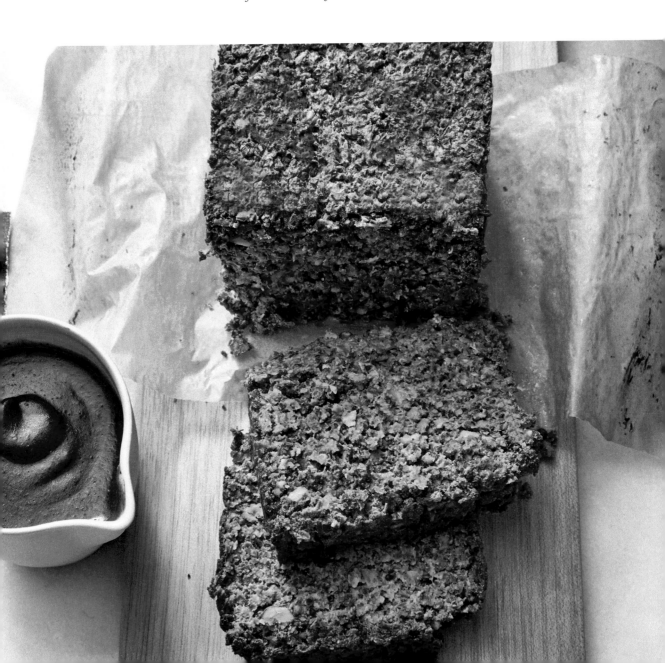

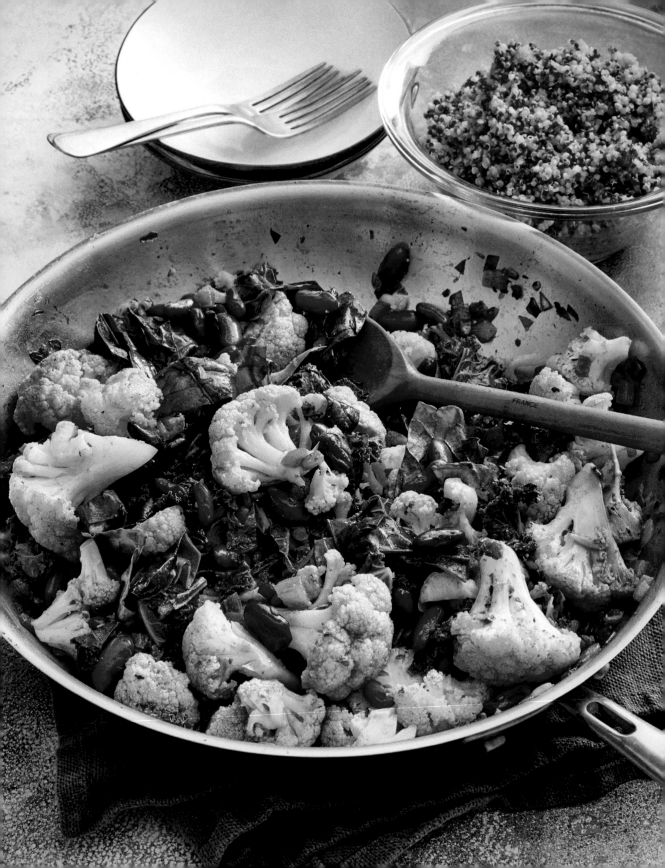

TURMERIC QUINOA AND RED BEANS WITH CAULIFLOWER AND CHARD

MAKES: *4 servings*   DIFFICULTY: *Easy*

This recipe takes less than thirty minutes to get on the table, thanks to quick-cooking quinoa.

1 cup/170g uncooked quinoa, well rinsed and drained

¾ teaspoon ground turmeric

2½ cups/620ml Light Vegetable Broth (page 214) or water

1 red onion, chopped

3 garlic cloves, finely chopped

3 cups/375g small cauliflower florets

1 teaspoon ground coriander

1 teaspoon smoked paprika

½ teaspoon dried thyme

½ teaspoon ground cumin

¼ teaspoon ground black pepper

¼ teaspoon red pepper flakes (optional)

1½ cups/260g cooked* or 1 (400g) BPA-free tin or Tetra Pak salt-free red kidney beans, drained and rinsed

8 ounces/225g chard, kale or spinach, tough stems removed, chopped

Combine the rinsed quinoa, turmeric and 2 cups/500ml of Light Vegetable Broth or water in a saucepan over a medium-high heat and bring to the boil. Lower the heat to a simmer and cook until the liquid is absorbed, about 15 minutes. Remove the saucepan from the heat, cover, and set aside for 5 minutes to allow the quinoa to steam. Uncover and fluff the quinoa with a fork. Set aside and keep warm.

While the quinoa is cooking, heat ¼ cup/60ml of water in a large saucepan over a medium heat. Add the onion and garlic and cook for 5 minutes to soften, stirring occasionally. Stir in the cauliflower, coriander, paprika, thyme, cumin, black pepper and red pepper flakes (if using). Add the kidney beans and ½ cup/120ml of Light Vegetable Broth and bring to the boil. Lower the heat to a simmer, cover, and cook for 8 minutes. Add the chard, stirring to wilt. Simmer until the vegetables are tender, about 5 minutes longer. To serve, spoon the quinoa into shallow bowls and top with the beans and vegetables. Serve hot.

*Turn to the Legumes and Grains Cooking Charts *on pages 218–221 for instruction, if needed.*

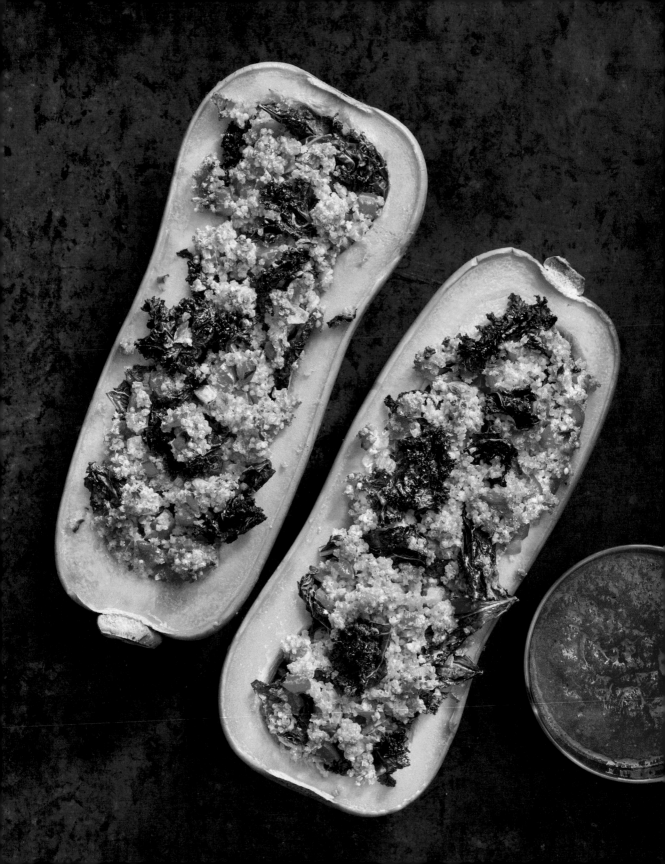

STUFFED WINTER SQUASH WITH MILLET AND KALE

MAKES: *2 to 4 servings*   DIFFICULTY: *Moderate*

To save time, make the stuffing while you pre-roast the squash, and prepare the sauce while the stuffed squash is baking. This recipe serves two as a main dish or four as a side dish.

SQUASH

1 kabocha or other large winter squash

STUFFING

1 red onion, chopped

2 garlic cloves, finely chopped

1 red pepper, de-seeded and chopped

1 tablespoon white miso paste

2 tablespoons nutritional yeast

1 teaspoon ground coriander

½ teaspoon ground cumin

¼ teaspoon cayenne

1 cup/200g uncooked millet

8 ounces/225g kale, tough stems removed, finely chopped

RED PEPPER–TOMATO SAUCE

¼ cup/40g finely chopped red onion

2 garlic cloves, finely chopped

2 plum tomatoes, cored and chopped

2 Roasted Red Peppers (page 217) or store-bought

1 teaspoon white miso paste

½ teaspoon dried thyme

1 (¼-inch/5mm) piece fresh turmeric, grated, or ¼ teaspoon ground

¼ teaspoon ground black pepper

Super-Charged Spice Blend (page 211)

FOR THE SQUASH: Preheat the oven to 200°C/400°F/gas mark 6. Line a large, rimmed roasting tin with a silicone mat or baking parchment.

Place the whole squash in the prepared tin and roast in the oven for about 20 minutes. Remove from the oven and set aside until cool enough to handle. Carefully remove the stem from the squash (it should be loose), and then cut the squash in half. Use a spoon to scoop out the seeds and fibres. Place the squash halves, cut side up, on the same roasting tin and set aside.

FOR THE STUFFING: While the squash is roasting, heat 2 cups/500ml of water in a large saucepan over a medium heat. Add the onion, garlic and pepper. Cook, stirring occasionally, until softened, about 5 minutes. Stir in the miso paste, nutritional yeast, coriander, cumin and cayenne. Add the millet and bring just to the boil. Lower the heat to low, cover, and cook for 10 minutes; then stir in the kale. Cover and continue to cook until the vegetables and millet are tender, 10 to 12 minutes longer. Remove from the heat, uncover, and allow to cool.

Fill the squash cavities with the millet mixture, packing them well. Cover and bake until the squash is tender, 30 to 40 minutes.

FOR THE SAUCE: While the squash is roasting, heat ¼ cup/60ml of water in a saucepan over a medium heat. Add the onion and garlic. Cover and cook for 4 minutes, or until soft. Stir in the chopped tomatoes, Roasted Red Peppers, miso paste, thyme, turmeric, black pepper and Super-Charged Spice Blend to taste. Cover and cook until the vegetables are very soft, about 5 minutes longer. Transfer to a blender or food processor and puree the sauce until smooth. Return the sauce to the saucepan and keep warm over a low heat until ready to use.

TO SERVE: Top the baked stuffed squash with the sauce and serve hot. If dividing into four servings, cut each squash half into two wedges.

SORGHUM AND CHICKPEAS WITH BROCCOLI AND TOMATOES

MAKES: *4 servings*   DIFFICULTY: *Easy*

The star of this dish is sorghum, a hearty and chewy grain that can be used in virtually any recipe calling for grains. If you want some variety, though, feel free to experiment with other whole grains when preparing this dish.

4 cups/1 litre Light Vegetable Broth (page 214)

1 cup/200g uncooked whole-grain sorghum

2 tablespoons Umami Sauce Redux (page 212)

1 tablespoon tahini

1 teaspoon white miso paste

1 teaspoon apple cider vinegar

¼ teaspoon cayenne

1 red onion, finely chopped

2 garlic cloves, finely chopped

3 cups/200g small broccoli florets

2 teaspoons grated fresh ginger

3 spring onions, finely chopped

1½ cups/250g cooked* or 1 (400g) BPA-free tin or Tetra Pak salt-free chickpeas, drained and rinsed

2 ripe plum tomatoes, cored and diced

Bring the Light Vegetable Broth to the boil in a saucepan over a high heat. Add the sorghum, cover with a tight-fitting lid, and lower the heat to a simmer. Cook for 45 minutes or until tender. Fluff with a fork, and then set aside.

In a small bowl, combine the Umami Sauce Redux, tahini, miso paste, apple cider vinegar and cayenne. Stir in ¼ cup/60ml of water and set aside.

Heat ¼ cup/60ml of water in a large skillet or wok over a medium-high heat. Add the onion and garlic and cook, stirring, until softened, about 5 minutes. Add the broccoli, ginger and spring onions and cook for 4 minutes. Stir in the chickpeas and tomatoes, then the umami sauce mixture; cook, stirring, until hot and well combined, about 5 minutes.

When ready to serve, combine the sorghum and the vegetable mixture and toss gently. Alternatively, spoon the sorghum into shallow bowls and top with the vegetable mixture. Serve hot.

Turn to the Legumes and Grains Cooking Charts *on pages 218–221 for instruction, if needed.*

WHAT ABOUT SORGHUM?

Gluten-free[77] sorghum pulls ahead of other grains for its fibre[78] and antioxidant power,[79] but its most exciting feature may be its resistant starch.

Most of its starch is slowly digested or fully resistant to digestion in the small intestine, providing prebiotics for your good gut flora.[80]

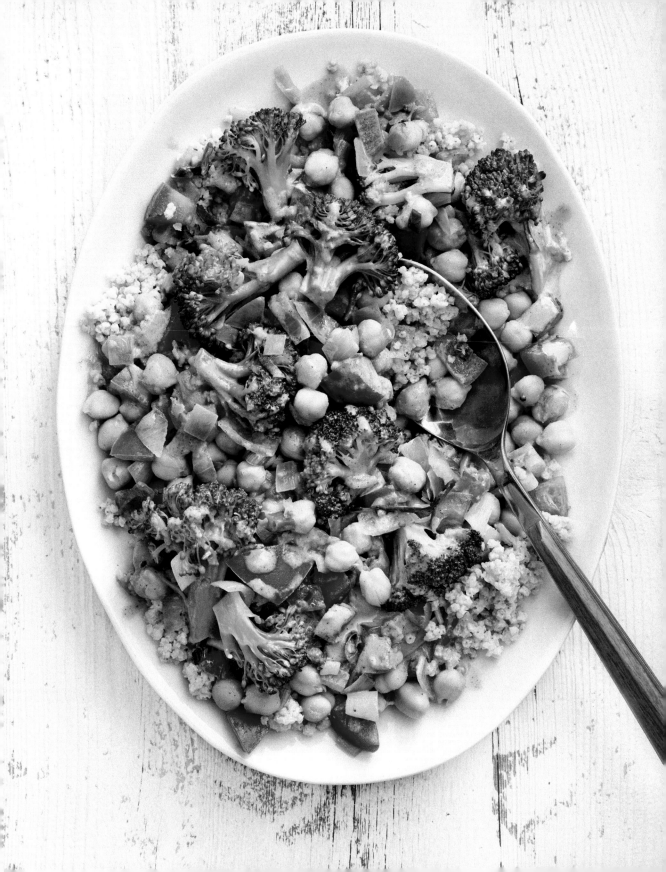

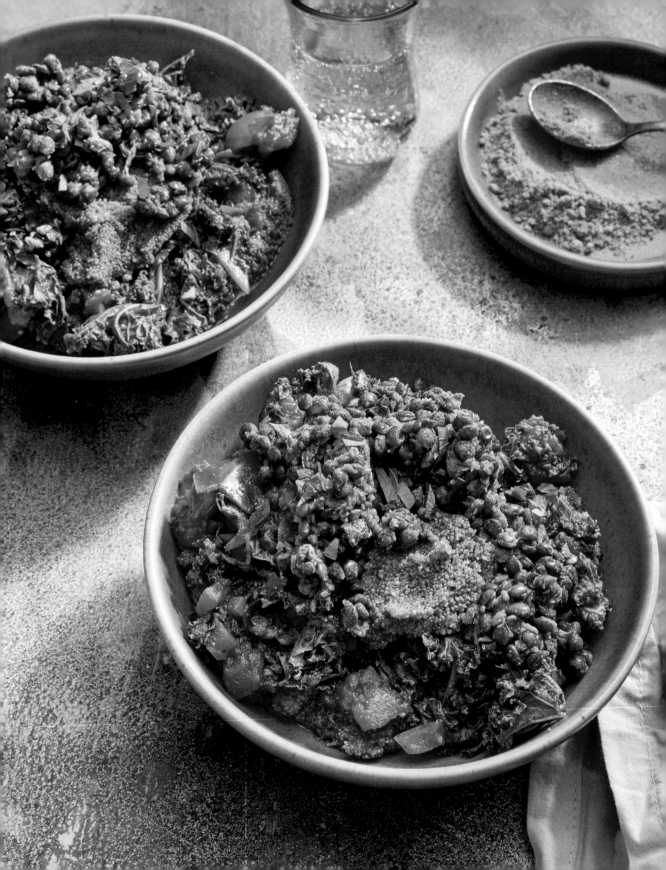

TEFF AND BLACK LENTILS OVER BERBERE-SPICED KALE

MAKES: *3 to 4 servings*   DIFFICULTY: *Moderate*

Teff is a fine grain about the size of a poppy seed. Naturally gluten-free and high in protein, it is a staple in many East African dishes. And berbere? It is a traditional Ethiopian spice blend available online or in well-stocked supermarkets. You can also make your own using the recipe on page 211.

LENTILS

1 cup/200g dried black lentils

1 teaspoon Berbere Spice Blend (page 211)

½ teaspoon onion powder

½ teaspoon garlic powder

TEFF

1 cup/195g uncooked teff

2 tablespoons nutritional yeast

1 teaspoon white miso paste

GREENS

1 cup/250ml Light Vegetable Broth (page 214)

1 red onion, chopped

2 garlic cloves, finely chopped

2 tablespoons salt-free tomato puree

2 teaspoons Berbere Spice Blend (page 211)

1 teaspoon smoked paprika

1 teaspoon ground coriander

1 (400g) BPA-free tin or Tetra Pak salt-free chopped tomatoes, undrained

8 cups/250g chopped kale or other dark leafy greens, tough stems removed

FOR THE LENTILS: In a small saucepan, combine the lentils, Berbere Spice Blend, onion powder and garlic powder. Add 2¼ cups/560ml of water and bring to a simmer. Cover and continue to simmer over a low heat until the lentils are tender but not mushy, about 20 minutes.

FOR THE TEFF: While the lentils are cooking, combine the teff, nutritional yeast and miso paste in another small saucepan. Stir in 1¼ cups/310ml of water and bring to a simmer. Lower the heat to low, cover and cook for 10 to 15 minutes, or until the teff is tender and the water is absorbed. Fluff it with a fork, cover and set aside until ready to serve.

FOR THE GREENS: Heat ¼ cup/60ml of the Light Vegetable Broth in a large skillet or heavy-based frying pan over a medium heat. Add the onion and garlic and cook until softened, about 5 minutes. Stir in the tomato puree, Berbere Spice Blend, paprika, coriander and tomatoes with their juices and bring to the boil. Lower the heat to a simmer; then add the kale and the remaining broth. Cook, stirring frequently, until the kale is tender and the flavours are combined, about 10 minutes.

TO SERVE: Divide the greens among three to four shallow bowls, top with the teff, followed by the lentils. Serve hot.

ARE ANCIENT GRAINS HEALTHIER?

Are ancient grains healthier than modern ones? Based on vitamin and mineral concentrations, it's pretty similar,[81] though primitive wheats have more antioxidant capacity.[82] Ancient wheat products do appear to be anti-inflammatory and may improve blood sugar control and cholesterol. The best available data suggest they're better, so if you have the choice, why not opt for ancient varieties?

GRAIN-STUFFED PEPPERS WITH CHEESY TOMATO SAUCE

MAKES: *4 servings*   DIFFICULTY: *Moderate*

This recipe calls for my beloved Basic BROL, the powerfully healthy and delicious combination of barley, rye, oats, and lentils, but any cooked whole grains may be used for the stuffing.

PEPPERS

4 large red peppers

1 red onion, finely chopped

3 garlic cloves, chopped

2 cups/360g Basic BROL (page 209), cooled, or other cooked* whole grains of your choice

1½ cups/250g cooked* or 1 (400g) BPA-free tin or Tetra Pak salt-free chickpeas, drained and rinsed

2 tablespoons ground flaxseeds

1 teaspoon white miso paste

¼ cup/35g nutritional yeast

4 tablespoons chopped fresh parsley

1 teaspoon smoked paprika

¼ teaspoon ground black pepper

1½ cups/390g tomato puree

CHEESY TOMATO SAUCE

1 cup/175g cooked* or BPA-free tinned or Tetra Pak salt-free white beans, drained and rinsed

⅓ cup/45g nutritional yeast

1 tablespoon apple cider vinegar

2 teaspoons fresh lemon juice

2 teaspoons white miso paste

½ teaspoon salt-free yellow mustard

½ teaspoon smoked paprika

½ teaspoon onion powder

1 (¼-inch/5mm) piece fresh turmeric, grated, or ¼ teaspoon ground

½ cup/130g tomato puree

FOR THE PEPPERS: Preheat the oven to 190°C/375°F/gas mark 5.

Cut off the top ½ inch/1cm of the peppers and set the tops aside. Remove the seeds from the pepper cavities and set the peppers aside. Chop the reserved pepper tops after discarding the stems. Heat ¼ cup/60ml of water in a large skillet or heavy-based frying pan over a medium-high heat. Add the chopped pepper tops, onion, and garlic and cook, stirring occasionally, until the onion is softened, about 7 minutes. Remove from the heat and set aside.

In a large bowl, combine the cooked and cooled Basic BROL, chickpeas, ground flaxseeds, miso paste, nutritional yeast, parsley, smoked paprika and black pepper. Stir in the cooked vegetables and ½ cup/130g of the tomato puree and mix well.

Fill the pepper cavities with the stuffing mixture. Arrange the stuffed peppers standing upright and next to one another in a baking dish. Pour the remaining tomato puree and ¼ cup/60ml of water around the peppers. Cover tightly and place in the oven. Bake for about 45 minutes, or until the peppers are soft and the stuffing is hot.

FOR THE CHEESY TOMATO SAUCE: While the peppers bake, make the sauce. Combine all the sauce ingredients, except the tomato puree, in a high-powered blender. Process until smooth, scraping down the sides as needed. Add the tomato puree and blend again. If the sauce is too thick, add a little water, 2 tablespoons at a time, until the sauce is smooth. Transfer the sauce to a saucepan and warm gently over a medium-low heat, stirring, to heat through. Taste and adjust the seasonings, if needed. Keep warm.

TO SERVE: When ready to serve, place each stuffed pepper upright on a serving plate or shallow serving bowl and top with the Cheesy Tomato Sauce.

Turn to the Legumes and Grains Cooking Charts on pages 218–221 for instruction, if needed.

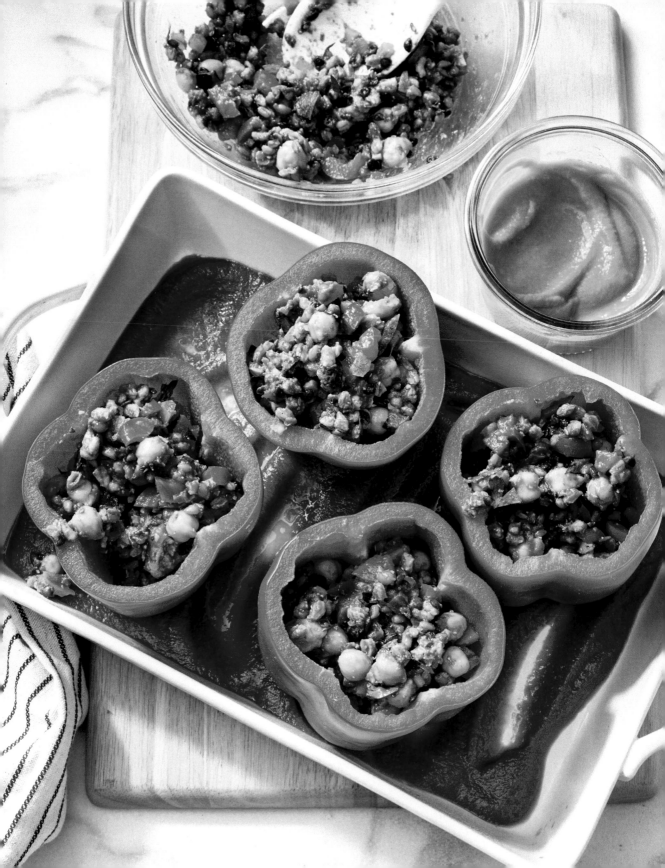

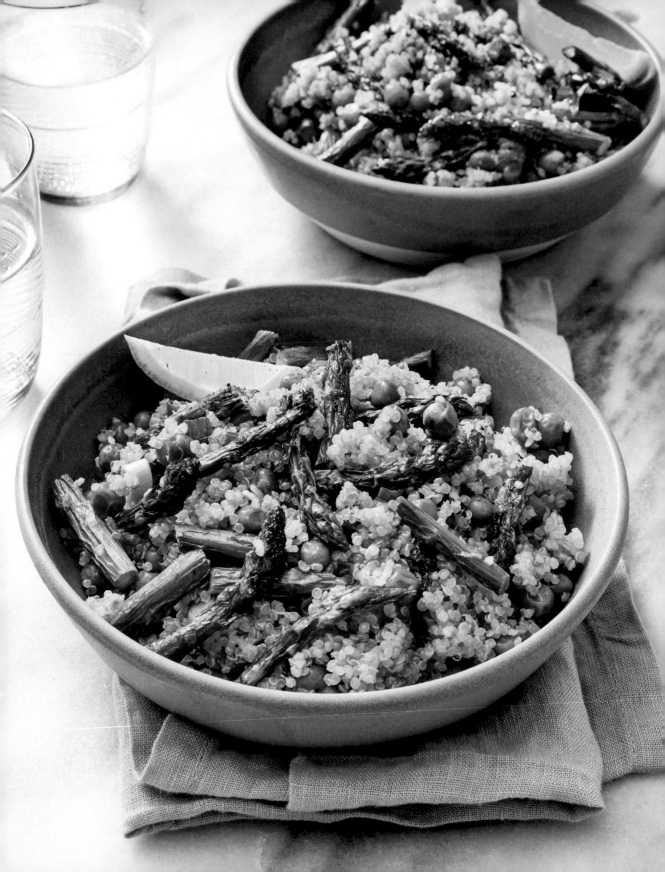

GREEN TEA QUINOA AND PEAS WITH ROASTED ASPARAGUS

MAKES: *4 servings*   DIFFICULTY: *Easy*

Inspired by the Japanese dish known as *ochazuke* (white rice steeped in green tea), this version uses quinoa instead of rice and pairs with roasted asparagus. Top with toasted nori and sesame seeds for even more texture and flavour.

3 green tea bags

3 cups/750ml hot water

1 pound/450g asparagus, trimmed and cut into 1-inch/2.5cm pieces

1 cup/170g uncooked quinoa, well rinsed and drained

1 garlic clove, finely chopped

1 teaspoon grated fresh ginger

1 cup/150g frozen peas

½ cup/75g finely chopped spring onions

2 tablespoons toasted sesame seeds

Ground black pepper

1 lemon, cut into wedges

Place the tea bags in a bowl with the hot water. Steep the tea for 8 to 10 minutes, then remove and discard the tea bags. Set the brewed tea aside.

Preheat the oven to 220°C/425°F/gas mark 7. Line a large, rimmed baking tray with a silicone mat or baking parchment.

Spread the asparagus pieces on the prepared baking tray. Roast in the oven for 10 to 15 minutes, or until tender and lightly browned on the edges. Set aside.

Combine the quinoa, garlic, ginger and steeped tea in a medium saucepan and bring to the boil. Lower the heat to medium-low, cover, and simmer for 10 minutes. Add the peas, cover, and cook for another 5 minutes, or until the tea is absorbed and the quinoa and peas are cooked. Remove from the heat and stir in the spring onions and asparagus.

To serve, spoon the quinoa into serving bowls and top with sesame seeds and black pepper. Serve with lemon wedges.

QUINOA AND TRIGLYCERIDES

Quinoa is a seed-like fruit high in protein,[83] vitamins, magnesium, iron, and zinc.[84] About a cup a day of cooked quinoa for twelve weeks led to a 36 per cent drop in triglycerides, comparable to what one gets with triglycerides-lowering drugs or high-dose fish oil supplements.[85]

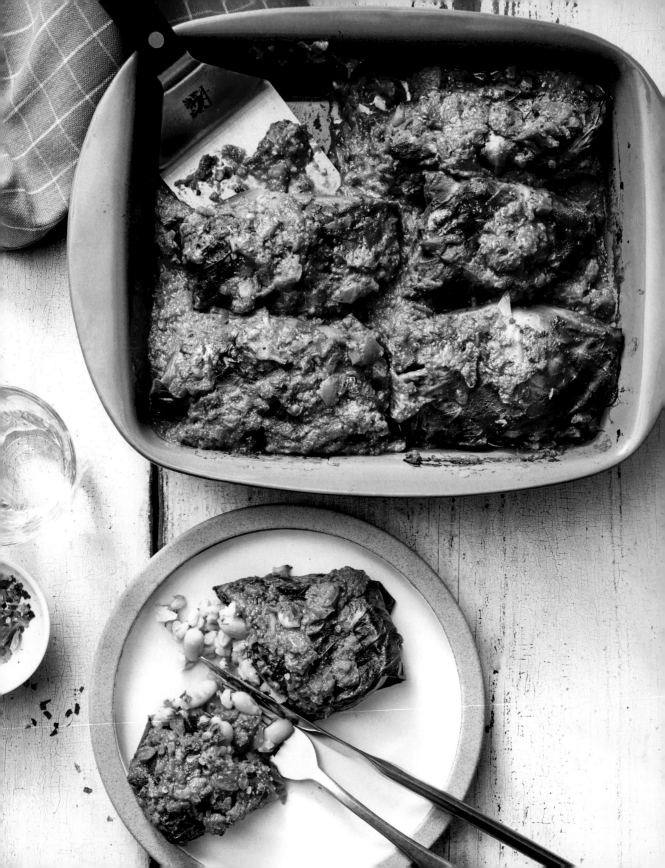

BARLEY-STUFFED CABBAGE ROLLS

MAKES: *4 servings*   DIFFICULTY: *Moderate*

Barley and cabbage go together like peanut butter and jam. These stuffed cabbage rolls are sure to become a favourite!

TOMATO SAUCE

½ cup/75g chopped onion

3 garlic cloves, finely chopped

2 teaspoons white miso paste

2 (400g) BPA-free tins or Tetra Paks salt-free finely chopped tomatoes

¼ cup/35g nutritional yeast

1 teaspoon dried oregano

1 teaspoon dried basil

¼ cup/4 tablespoons chopped fresh parsley

Ground black pepper

FILLING

2 cups/370g cooked* barley

3 cups/525g cooked* or 2 (400g) BPA-free tins or Tetra Paks salt-free white beans, drained and rinsed

1 small red onion, finely chopped

2 garlic cloves, finely chopped

2 tablespoons nutritional yeast

1 teaspoon white miso paste

¼ cup/4 tablespoons finely chopped fresh parsley

1 teaspoon smoked paprika

Ground black pepper

CABBAGE

1 large head red cabbage

FOR THE TOMATO SAUCE: Heat ¼ cup/60ml of water in a large saucepan over a medium heat. Add the onion and garlic and cook, stirring occasionally, until the onion is tender, about 5 minutes. Stir in the miso paste, tomatoes, nutritional yeast, oregano, basil, parsley and black pepper to taste. Lower the heat to low, cover, and cook until the flavours are well blended, about 20 minutes. Taste and adjust the seasonings, if needed. Set aside.

FOR THE FILLING: In a bowl, combine all the filling ingredients and mix well. Set aside.

Preheat the oven to 190°C/375°F/gas mark 5.

FOR THE CABBAGE: Trim the cabbage of any damaged leaves and use a sharp knife to cut out the core. Place the cabbage, cut side down, in a large pot along with enough water to cover, and then bring to the boil. Cook until the leaves soften and begin to unfold, about 10 minutes. Use tongs to remove the leaves as soon as they soften and carefully place them on a plate to cool. Continue until you have at least 12 cooked leaves.

One at a time, arrange the leaves on a cutting board with the stem end nearest you. Place about ¼ cup/4 ` of filling at the stem end. Fold the stem end and sides over the filling and roll the cabbage leaf up tightly. Continue until all the cabbage rolls have been made.

TO ASSEMBLE AND SERVE: Spread half of the sauce onto the bottom of a large, shallow baking dish. Arrange the cabbage rolls, seam side down, on top of the sauce. Spoon all but 1 cup of sauce over the cabbage rolls, and then cover the rolls with 3 to 4 leftover leaves. Spoon the remaining sauce over the leaves. Cover the baking dish tightly and bake for 45 minutes, or until the rolls are tender. Serve hot.

Turn to the Legumes and Grains Cooking Charts *on pages 218–221 for instruction, if needed.*

7
BREAKFAST

Is breakfast the most important meal of the day? Well, according to chronobiology, the study
of how our body's natural cycles – mental, physical and emotional – are affected by the
rhythms of the sun, moon and seasons, it seems that it is when it comes to losing weight.
Calories eaten in the morning seem to be less fattening than calories eaten in the evening. More
calories are burned off in the morning due to diet-induced thermogenesis, the amount of energy the
body takes to digest and process a meal, given off in part as waste heat. When people consume
the exact same meal in the morning, afternoon, and at night, their body uses up about 25 per cent
more calories to process the meal in the afternoon than at night and about 50 per cent more calories
to digest it in the morning.[86] That leaves fewer net calories in the morning to be stored as fat.
These bright, bountiful breakfast recipes will help you heed the proverb 'Eat breakfast
like a king, lunch like a prince, and dinner like a pauper' and take advantage of
the metabolic benefits to distributing more calories to earlier in the day.

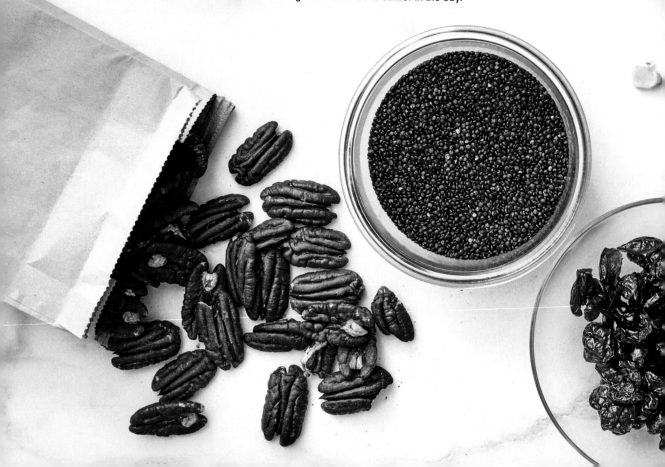

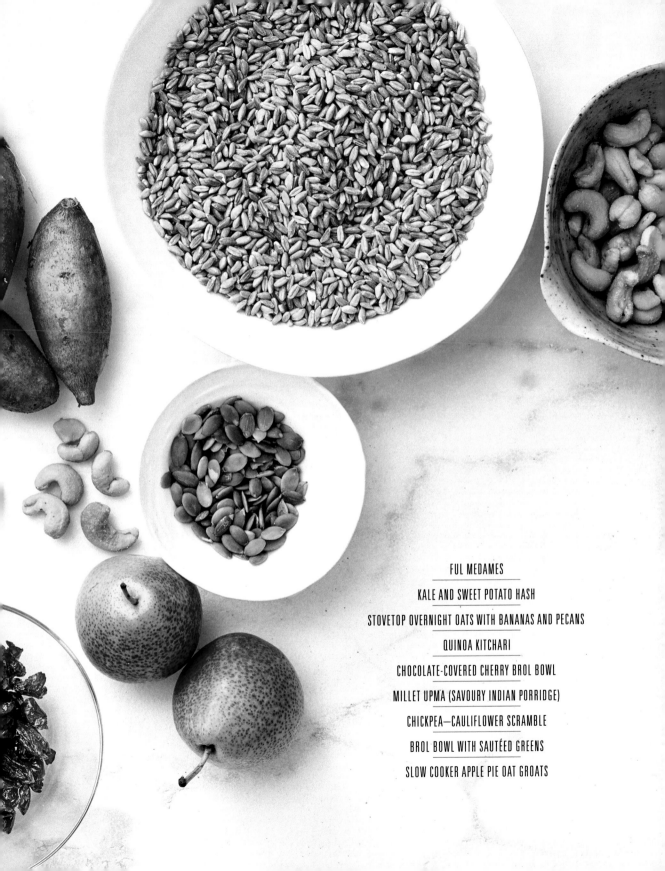

FUL MEDAMES

MAKES: *3 to 4 servings*   DIFFICULTY: *Easy*

This stewed broad bean dish is popular for breakfast in Egypt. For an even heartier meal, serve it over hummus.

BEANS

½ cup/120ml Light Vegetable Broth (page 214)

1 small red onion, finely chopped

3 Roasted Garlic (page 216) cloves, finely chopped

1 cup/200g coarsely chopped tomato

1 teaspoon white miso paste

1 teaspoon ground cumin

½ teaspoon paprika

¼ teaspoon ground black pepper

3–4 cups/510–680g cooked* broad beans

2 tablespoons fresh lemon juice

GARNISH

½ cup/75g chopped cucumber

½ cup/100g chopped ripe tomato

¼ cup/4 tablespoons finely chopped fresh parsley

½ teaspoon dried oregano

1 tablespoon fresh lemon juice

Ground black pepper

TO SERVE

Coarsely ground nigella seeds

FOR THE BEANS: Heat the Light Vegetable Broth in a saucepan over a medium heat. Add the onion, cover, and cook until softened, about 5 minutes, stirring occasionally. Add the Roasted Garlic, tomato, miso paste, cumin, paprika and black pepper. Cook, stirring, for about 2 minutes to blend the flavours. Stir in the cooked broad beans and cook for 5 minutes to heat through. Stir in the lemon juice and keep warm.

FOR THE GARNISH: In a bowl, combine all the garnish ingredients, including black pepper to taste, and mix well.

TO SERVE: Spoon the broad bean mixture into bowls and top with the mixed garnish. Sprinkle with nigella seeds and serve.

＊*Turn to the* Legumes and Grains Cooking Charts *on pages 218–221 for instruction, if needed.*

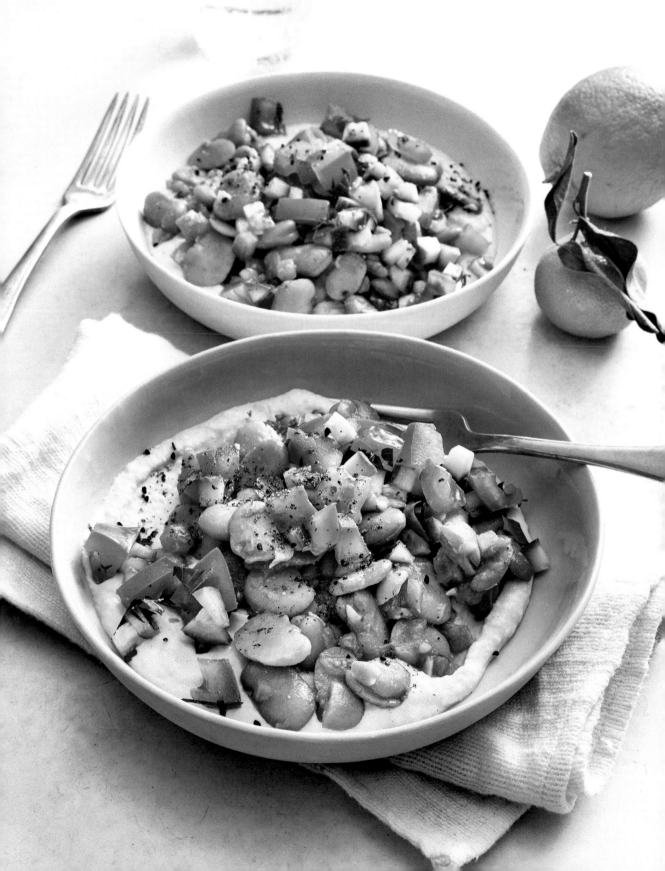

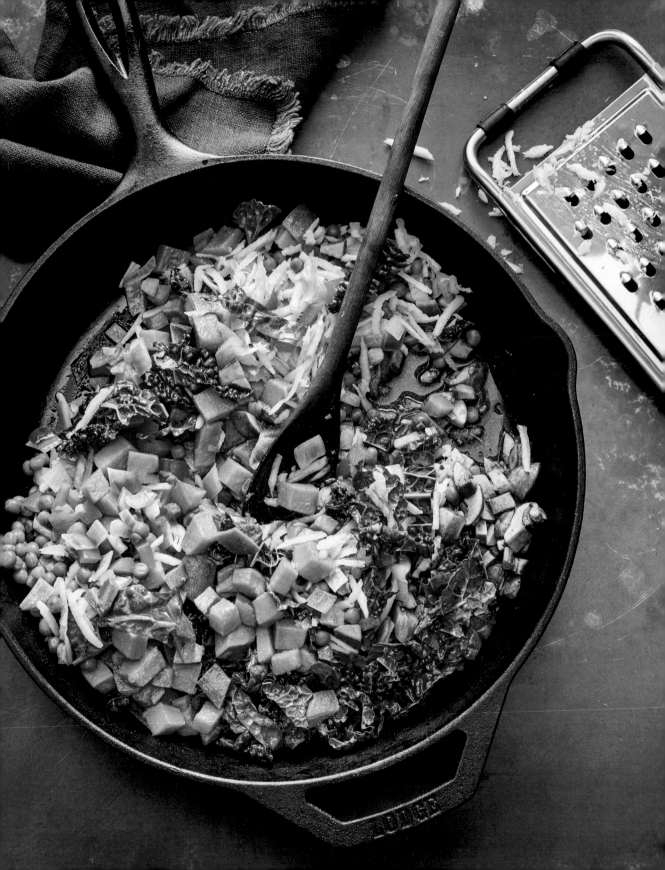

CAVOLO NERO AND SWEET POTATO HASH

MAKES: *4 servings*   DIFFICULTY: *Easy*

A hearty hash is a great way to start the day. If I know I'll be rushed in the morning, I prep the ingredients the night before or use leftover cooked ingredients. If I know I'll be super rushed, I make the entire recipe ahead of time and then simply heat and enjoy.

1 large sweet potato, diced

1 large red onion, finely chopped

1 parsnip, grated

1 small red pepper, de-seeded and chopped

4 ounces/115g baby portobello mushrooms, chopped

2 tablespoons Umami Sauce Redux (page 212)

6 ounces/175g cavolo nero, tough stems removed, coarsely chopped

½ cup/75g fresh or thawed frozen peas

Ground black pepper

Salt-Free Hot Sauce (page 216) (optional)

Preheat the oven to 220°C/425°F/gas mark 7. Line a baking tray with a silicone mat or baking parchment.

Spread the diced sweet potato in a single layer on the prepared tray. Roast in the oven for 30 minutes, or until tender, stirring about half-way through. Remove from the oven and set aside.

Heat ¼ cup/60ml of water in a large skillet or heavy-based frying pan over a medium-high heat. Add the onion, parsnip and pepper and cook until softened, about 5 minutes. Add the mushrooms and Umami Sauce Redux and cook, stirring, for 1 minute longer. Stir in the cavolo nero, peas and black pepper to taste. Cook until the cavolo nero is wilted and tender, about 4 minutes. Drain off any liquid from the skillet; then add the roasted sweet potato and cook, pressing down with a metal spatula to lightly mash the ingredients together. Cook for 5 minutes, or until lightly browned on the bottom, then turn the hash with a metal spatula to lightly brown on the other side. Serve hot with Salt-Free Hot Sauce (if using).

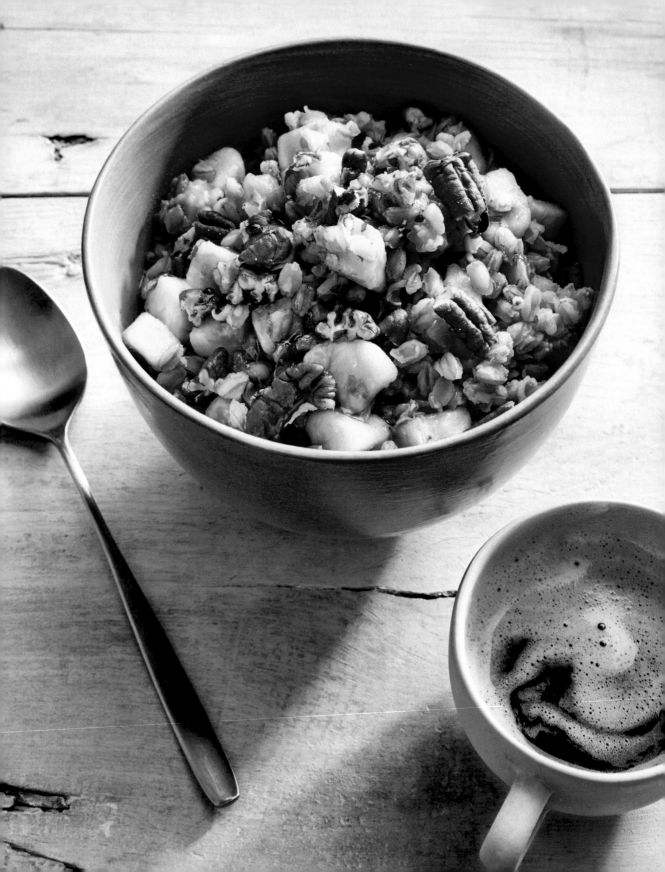

STOVETOP OVERNIGHT OATS WITH BANANAS AND PECANS

MAKES: *4 servings*   DIFFICULTY: *Easy*

These overnight oat groats, also known as groatmeal, are a quick and easy way to have a hearty, flavoursome breakfast.

1 cup/180g oat groats

2 ripe bananas

¼ teaspoon ground nutmeg

2 tablespoons chopped pecans

Date Syrup (page 217) (optional)

The night before, bring 2 cups/500ml of water to the boil in a medium saucepan. Add the oat groats, cover, and return to the boil for 2 minutes. Remove the pan from the heat. Set aside, covered, until morning.

The next morning, return the covered saucepan to the stovetop. Remove the lid and cook over a medium heat, stirring occasionally, for 6 to 8 minutes, or until the oats are tender and heated through. If all the water is absorbed before the oats become tender, add up to ½ cup/120ml of additional water and continue to cook while stirring occasionally for a few more minutes until tender.

Peel and chop the bananas and add to the oats along with the nutmeg. Cook, stirring, over a low heat for 1 to 2 minutes to combine and blend the flavours. To serve, spoon into serving bowls and sprinkle with chopped pecans and a swirl of Date Syrup (if using).

It's all about you! Customize your morning oat groats – a.k.a. groatmeal – with any combination of these toppings to satisfy your palate: sliced bananas, blueberries, strawberries, raspberries, blackberries, chopped peaches, chopped mango, slivered almonds, chopped pecans, chopped walnuts, sunflower seeds, pumpkin seeds, chia seeds, hemp seeds, cacao nibs, ground flaxseeds, dried goji berries, dried cranberries, ground cinnamon, mixed spice, ground nutmeg and any other whole food goodness that tickles your fancy!

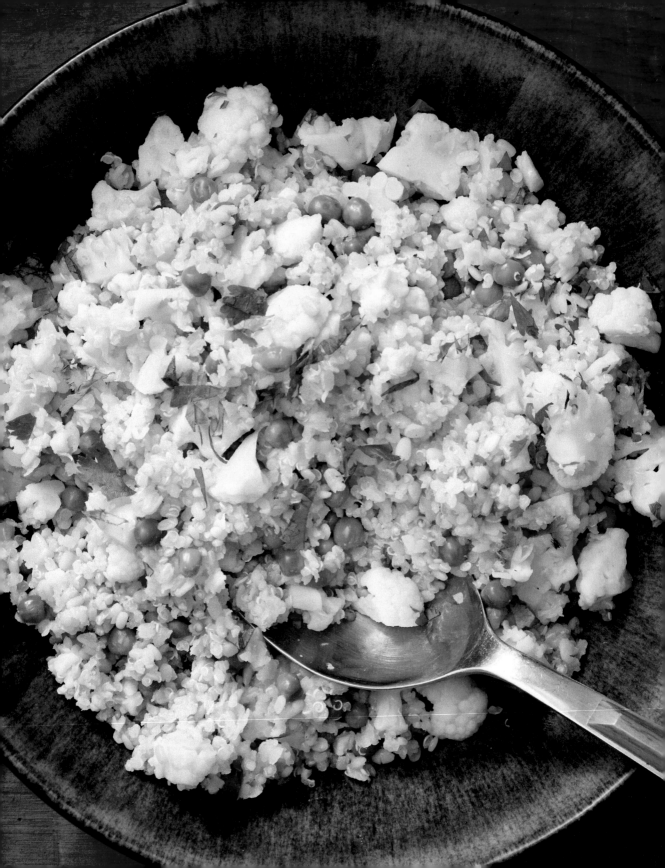

QUINOA KITCHARI

MAKES: *4 servings*   DIFFICULTY: *Easy*

Quinoa stands in for basmati rice in this savoury Indian breakfast porridge. Feel free to swap in different vegetables for the cauliflower and peas, according to your preference or what you have on hand.

½ cup/100g moong dal (split yellow mung beans)

½ cup/85g uncooked quinoa, well rinsed and drained

1 cup/125g small-chopped cauliflower

½ cup/75g peas

2 teaspoons grated fresh ginger

1 teaspoon ground coriander

½ teaspoon ground cumin

1 (½-inch/1cm) piece fresh turmeric, grated, or ½ teaspoon ground

1 teaspoon white miso paste

¼ teaspoon ground black pepper

½ cup/4 tablespoons chopped fresh coriander

1 lemon, cut into wedges

Soak the moong dal in enough water to cover for 15 minutes, then drain and rinse.

In a saucepan, combine the moong dal and quinoa with 4 cups/ 1 litre of water. Bring to the boil over a medium-high heat, then lower the heat to a low simmer and cook, stirring occasionally, for about 20 minutes. Stir in the cauliflower and peas, then cook for 5 minutes longer, or until the consistency of the dal is soft and creamy.

Stir in the ginger, coriander, cumin, turmeric, miso paste and black pepper. Cook for 5 minutes longer, stirring, to heat through. Remove from the heat and allow to sit for 5 minutes for the flavours to blend. Taste and adjust the seasoning, if needed, and stir again. Top with the coriander and serve with lemon wedges.

CHOCOLATE-COVERED CHERRY BROL BOWL

MAKES: *1 serving*   DIFFICULTY: *Easy*

A chocolatey and fruity breakfast with all the benefits of savoury whole grains? Yes, please!

1 cup/180g cooked Basic BROL (page 209), warmed

1 tablespoon unsweetened cocoa powder

1 tablespoon Date Syrup (page 217) or treacle

2 tablespoons walnut pieces

½ cup/115g fresh pitted or thawed frozen dark cherries

Spoon the Basic BROL into a bowl. Sprinkle with the cocoa, then drizzle with Date Syrup. Add the walnuts and half of the cherries. Stir together until combined. Top with the remaining cherries and serve.

CEREAL OR OATMEAL?

After eating Honey Nut Cheerios, study participants felt significantly hungrier than after the same calories of oatmeal. Food structure, not just nutrient composition, may be critical for optimal health.[87] Rolled oats, for instance, have a lower glycemic index than instant oatmeal,[88] and oat flakes cause lower blood sugar and insulin spikes than powdered oats.[89] Different forms of the same ingredient can have different effects.

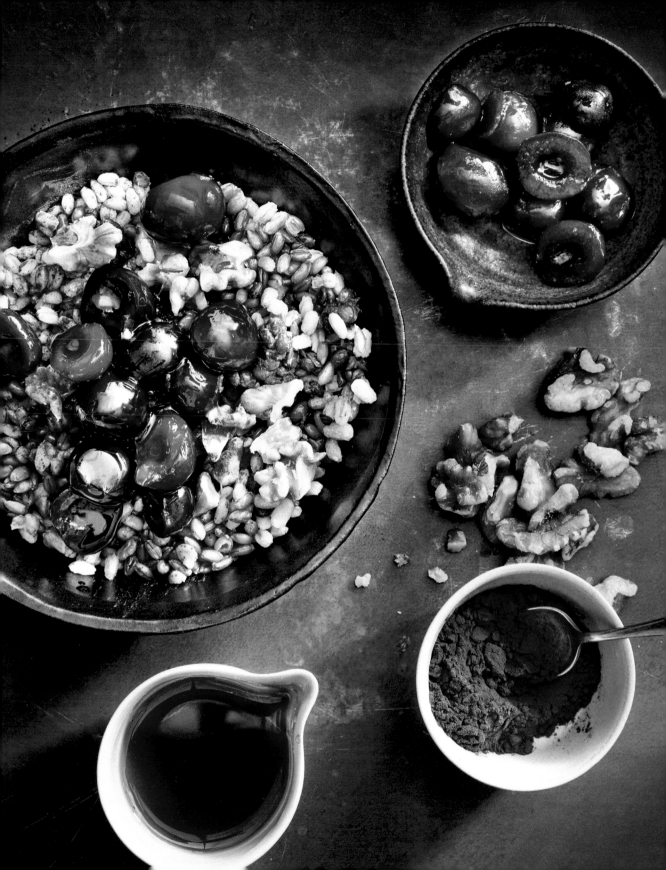

MILLET UPMA
(SAVOURY INDIAN PORRIDGE)

MAKES: *4 servings*   DIFFICULTY: *Easy*

If you're looking for something different to wake up your taste buds in the morning, try this savoury Indian porridge. This version of upma is made with millet because it's a quick-cooking grain, but you can use another whole grain, such as quinoa, if you prefer. If using a longer-cooking grain, adjust the cooking time accordingly.

1 red onion, chopped

1 carrot, finely chopped

2 teaspoons grated fresh ginger

1 green chilli, finely chopped (optional)

1 (½-inch/1cm) piece of fresh turmeric, grated, or ½ teaspoon ground

1¼ teaspoons garam masala, or to taste

1 teaspoon ground coriander

½ teaspoon ground cumin

1 teaspoon white miso paste

½ cup/75g frozen peas

1 plum tomato, cored and chopped

1 cup/200g uncooked millet, rinsed and drained

2 cups/500ml Light Vegetable Broth (page 214) or water

2 teaspoons fresh lemon juice

2 tablespoons cashew pieces

2 tablespoons finely chopped fresh coriander

Heat ¼ cup/60ml of water in a large saucepan over a medium heat. Add the onion, carrot, ginger and chilli (if using) and cook for 5 minutes to soften. Stir in the turmeric, garam masala, coriander, cumin and miso paste, then add the peas and tomato. Stir in the millet, then add the Light Vegetable Broth and bring to the boil.

Lower the heat to low, cover, and cook for 20 minutes, or until the millet is tender. Remove from the heat and set aside, covered, for about 8 minutes. Uncover, add the lemon juice, and fluff the millet with a fork. Spoon the upma into bowls and top with the cashews and coriander. Serve hot.

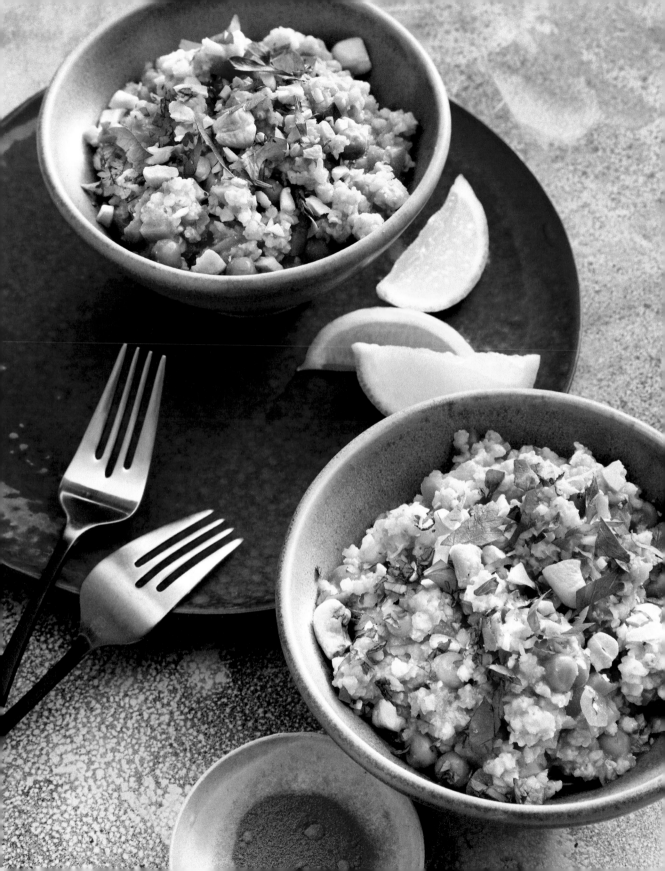

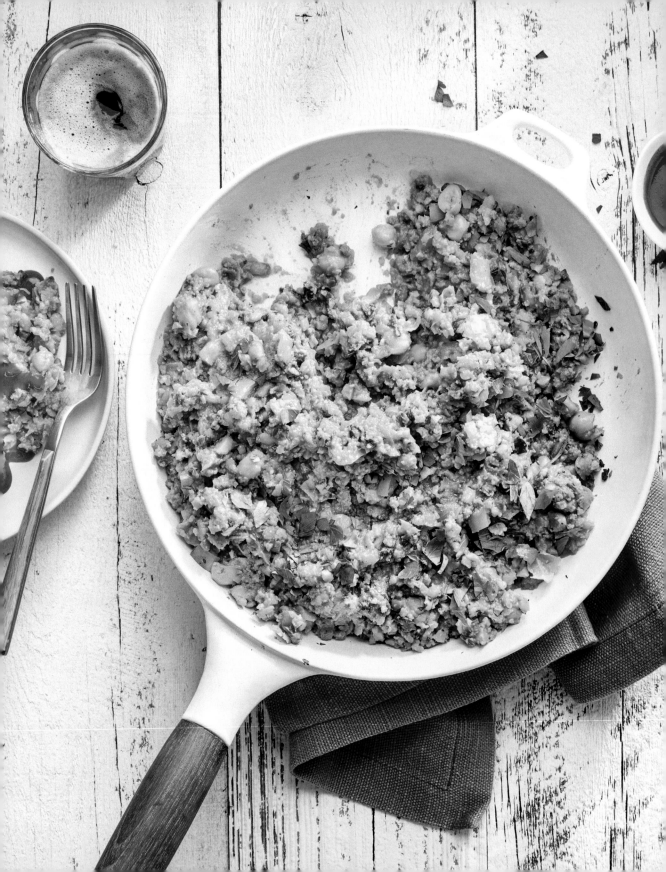

CHICKPEA–CAULIFLOWER SCRAMBLE

MAKES: *4 servings*   DIFFICULTY: *Easy*

Although this dish is in the breakfast section, grated cauliflower and mashed chickpeas combine to make a hearty and delicious scramble that's good any time of day. Top it with Fresh Tomato Salsa (page 210), Salt-Free Hot Sauce (page 216), or Cheesy Tomato Sauce (page 162) for extra oomph.

1 small onion, chopped

1 red or yellow pepper, de-seeded and chopped

3 cups/350g grated cauliflower

8 ounces/225g mushrooms, coarsely chopped

¼ cup/35g nutritional yeast

2½ teaspoons Dr Greger's Special Spice Blend (page 212)

½ teaspoon ground turmeric

1½ cups/250g cooked* or 1 (400g) BPA-free tin or Tetra Pak salt-free chickpeas, drained and rinsed

2 tablespoons finely chopped fresh parsley

Heat ¼ cup/60ml of water in a large skillet or heavy-based frying pan over a medium heat. Add the onion, cover, and cook until tender, about 5 minutes. Add the pepper and cauliflower; then cover and cook, stirring occasionally, until tender, about 5 minutes. Stir in the mushrooms, nutritional yeast, Dr Greger's Special Spice Blend, and turmeric. Cover and cook for 5 minutes.

While the veggies are cooking, mash the chickpeas and add them to the skillet. Cover and cook, stirring occasionally, until heated through and any liquid is absorbed, about 5 minutes longer.

Top with the parsley and any optional topping you prefer (see recipe introduction above), and serve hot.

*Turn to the Legumes and Grains Cooking Charts *on pages 218–221 for instruction, if needed.*

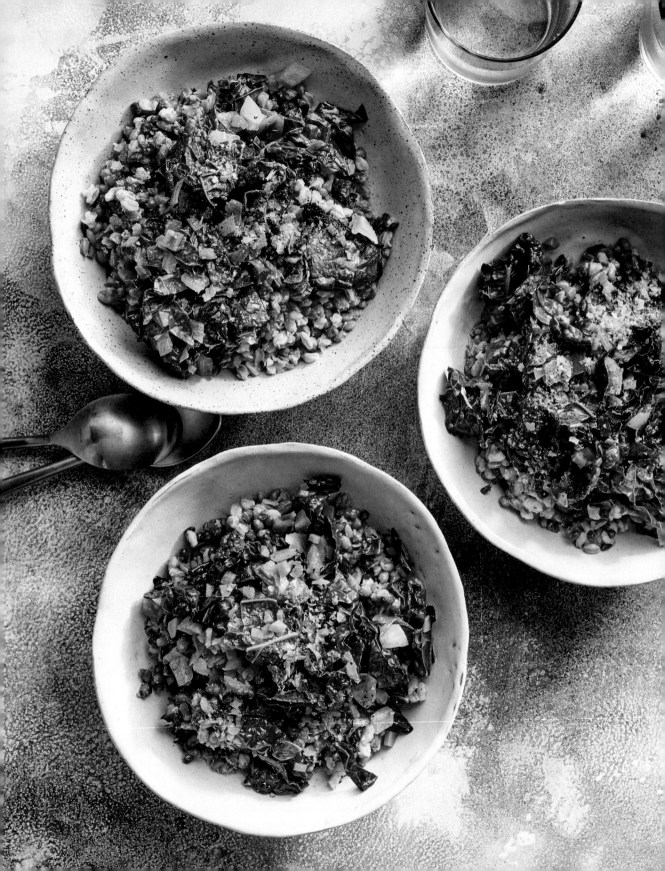

BROL BOWL WITH SAUTÉED GREENS

MAKES: *1 serving*   DIFFICULTY: *Easy*

Savoury breakfast lovers, rejoice! This dish reheats well, whether in a microwave or on the stovetop, so consider making extra portions. Store them in airtight containers in your fridge so you can have an amazing breakfast almost instantly.

½ cup/120ml Light Vegetable Broth (page 214)

½ cup/75g finely chopped red onion

1 garlic clove, finely chopped

1 small carrot, finely chopped

1 teaspoon white miso paste

6 ounces/175g cavolo nero, tough stems removed, coarsely chopped

1 cup/180g cooked Basic BROL (page 209), warmed

1 tablespoon nutritional yeast

Ground black pepper

1 lemon, cut into wedges

Heat the Light Vegetable Broth in a medium skillet or heavy-based frying pan over a medium heat. Add the onion, garlic and carrot and cook, stirring, until the vegetables are softened, about 7 minutes. Stir in the miso paste and cavolo nero and cook, stirring, until the cavolo nero is wilted and tender, about 4 minutes. Drain off any remaining liquid.

To serve, spoon the warmed Basic BROL into a bowl. Sprinkle with the nutritional yeast and black pepper to taste. Top with the hot cavolo nero mixture and serve with lemon wedges.

ARE MICROWAVE OVENS SAFE?

A famous radio telescope scanning the cosmos for extraterrestrial civilizations detected 'fast radio bursts'. Signs of extragalactic intelligence? No. It turns out ET was a microwave in the staff cafeteria that the telescope picked up when someone opened the door.[90] Indeed, there is some leakage of microwaves during operation,[91] but it appears microwaves should be safe – though it can't hurt to stand back when they're in operation.

SLOW COOKER APPLE PIE OAT GROATS

MAKES: *4 servings*   DIFFICULTY: *Easy*

Waking up to the sweet, rich aroma of this apple pie-inspired groatmeal is a great inducement to getting out of bed in the morning. This dish needs about eight hours for the oat groats to soak and another eight hours for the groatmeal to cook in a slow cooker, so plan ahead. The effort is minimal, and the time is very well worth it.

---

1 cup/180g oat groats, soaked for about 8 hours in water and then drained

2 tablespoons ground chia seeds

1 teaspoon ground cinnamon

1 apple, cored and grated with its peel

Optional toppings: goji berries, Date Syrup (page 217), ground cinnamon, dried or fresh fruit, or sliced or chopped nuts

In a 3.8 litre (or larger) slow cooker, combine the drained soaked oat groats with the chia seeds and cinnamon, stirring to mix well. Add the grated apple and 2¾ cups/675ml of water and stir to combine. Put the lid on the slow cooker and cook on low for about 8 hours. Stir the cooked groatmeal before spooning into serving bowls. Sprinkle with your desired toppings and serve.

DON'T PEEL YOUR APPLES

Eating just one apple a day is associated with a 35 per cent lower risk of dying from all causes.[92] Flavonoids, phytonutrients concentrated in the skins of apples, may play a role by improving artery function,[93] so don't peel your apples!

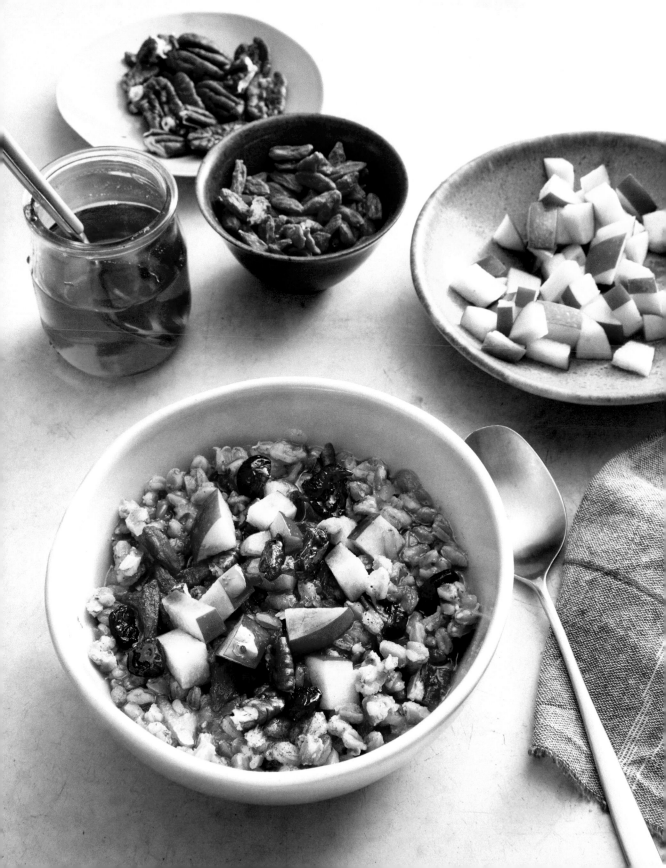

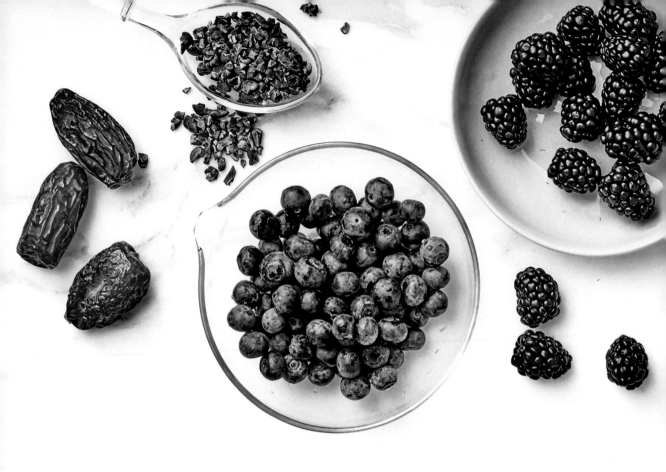

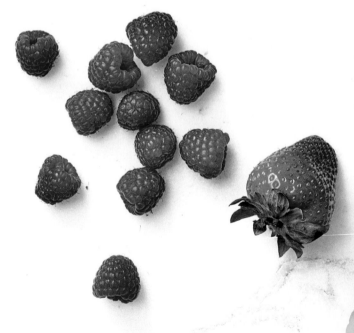

FRESH BERRIES WITH CHOCOLATE BALSAMIC SYRUP

STONE FRUIT BOWLS

MANGO—RASPBERRY CHIA PUDDING

CRUST-FREE PUMPKIN PIE

BLACK FOREST CHIA PUDDING

BAKED APPLES WITH WALNUTS AND GOJI BERRIES

TROPICAL SMOOTHIE BOWLS

GINGER ROASTED PEARS

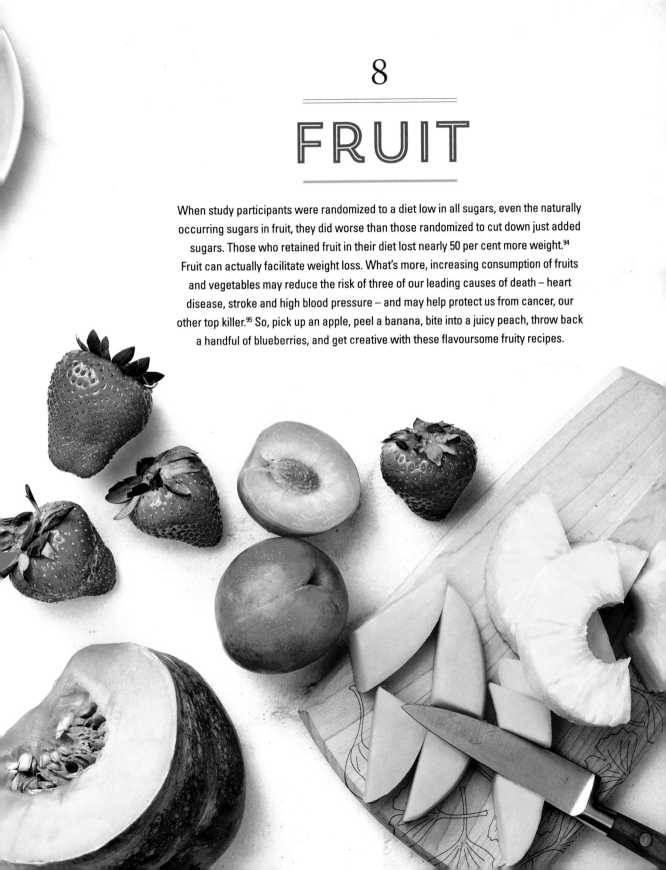

8

FRUIT

When study participants were randomized to a diet low in all sugars, even the naturally occurring sugars in fruit, they did worse than those randomized to cut down just added sugars. Those who retained fruit in their diet lost nearly 50 per cent more weight.[94] Fruit can actually facilitate weight loss. What's more, increasing consumption of fruits and vegetables may reduce the risk of three of our leading causes of death – heart disease, stroke and high blood pressure – and may help protect us from cancer, our other top killer.[95] So, pick up an apple, peel a banana, bite into a juicy peach, throw back a handful of blueberries, and get creative with these flavoursome fruity recipes.

FRESH BERRIES WITH CHOCOLATE BALSAMIC SYRUP

MAKES: *4 servings*   DIFFICULTY: *Easy*

Make this quick and easy treat at the peak of berry season. I like to combine several different berries, but it's also delicious with just one or two types, if you prefer. This recipe serves four, but if you're making it for just one or two people, cut back on the amount of berries and/or only add the mint leaves and balsamic when ready to serve.

⅓ cup/75ml chocolate balsamic vinegar or Balsamic Syrup (page 215)

1½ cups/225g strawberries, hulled and halved

¾ cup/95g raspberries

1 cup/100g blueberries

½ cup/75g blackberries

2 tablespoons fresh mint leaves

1 tablespoon cacao nibs

¼ cup/30g coarsely chopped pecans or walnuts (optional)

If not using Balsamic Syrup, pour the chocolate balsamic vinegar into a small saucepan and simmer over low heat for about 10 minutes, or until reduced by about one-third. Remove from the heat and set the vinegar aside to cool to room temperature before using.

In a large serving bowl, combine all the berries with the mint leaves. Spoon into individual glass serving bowls and drizzle on the chocolate balsamic reduction or Balsamic Syrup. Top with the cacao nibs and nuts (if using).

BENEFITS OF BLUEBERRIES ON HEART DISEASE AND CHOLESTEROL

Four out of five studies suggest that increased intake of berries, with their brightly coloured pigments called anthocyanins, is significantly associated with a reduction in risk of coronary heart disease, our number one killer, by 12 to 32 per cent.[96]

What do berries have to do with the heart?

Berries help control bad LDL cholesterol, blood pressure, blood sugars, body weight, diabetes, and inflammation.[97]

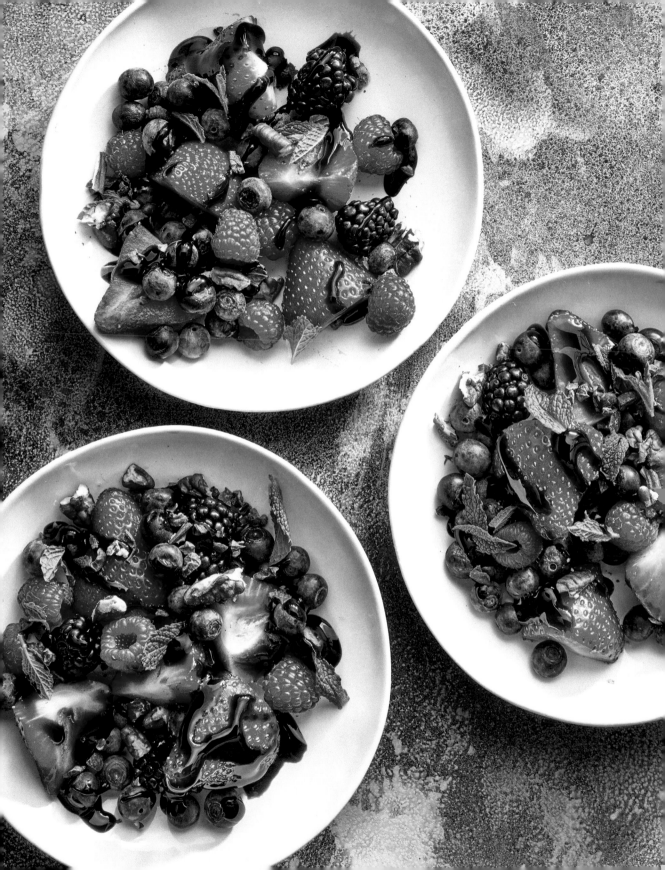

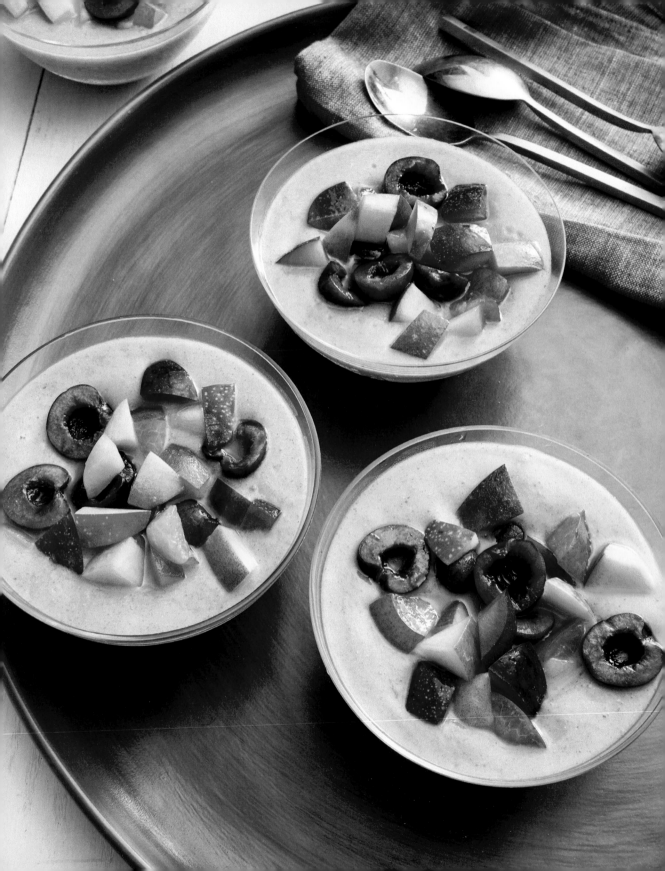

STONE FRUIT BOWLS

MAKES: *4 servings*   DIFFICULTY: *Easy*

A drupe, more commonly known as stone fruit, is so named because it contains a stone (or pit) inside. Many popular stone fruits, such as cherries, plums, peaches, nectarines, mangoes and dates, are in season in late summer.

3 tablespoons ground chia seeds

1½ cups/260g fresh or thawed frozen diced mango

1 teaspoon fresh lemon juice

2 pitted soft dates, soaked for 10 minutes in hot water and then drained

3 ripe apricots, pitted and quartered

3 ripe plums, pitted and cut into 1-inch/2.5cm pieces

2 ripe peaches or nectarines, pitted and cut into 1-inch/2.5cm pieces

2 cups/450g pitted cherries

In a small bowl, combine the chia seeds and ¼ cup/60ml of water and mix well. Set aside for 10 minutes to thicken.

In a food processor or blender, combine the mango, lemon juice, dates and the chia mixture and process until smooth. Divide equally among four small glass dessert bowls. Cover and refrigerate until firm, 4 hours or overnight.

Combine the apricots, plums, peaches, and cherries in a large bowl. Toss gently to combine.

To serve, spoon the fruit evenly over the chilled mango mixture. Serve immediately.

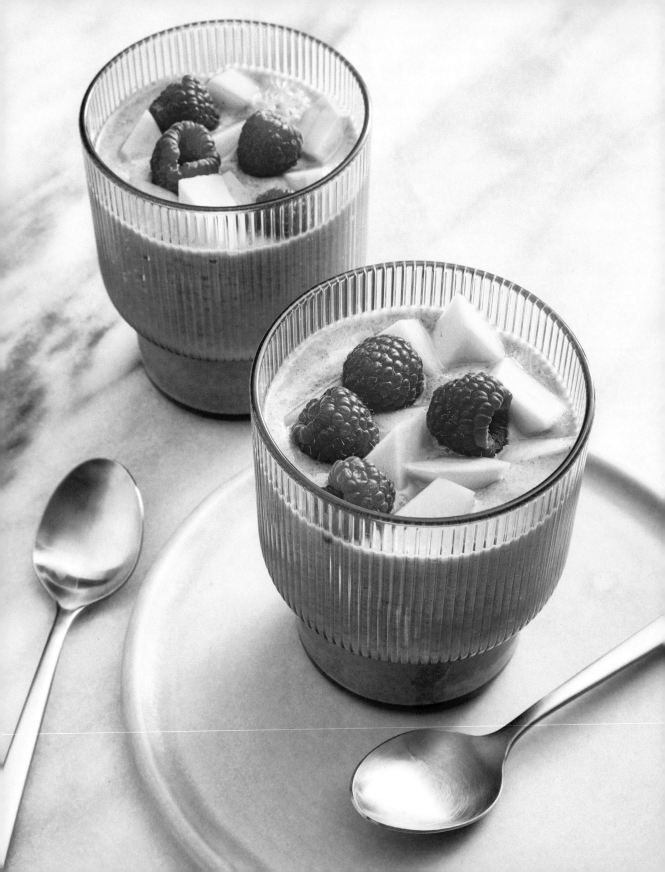

MANGO-RASPBERRY CHIA PUDDING

MAKES: *2 servings*   DIFFICULTY: *Easy*

This refreshing chia pudding can be made with different fruits whether to take advantage of the fruits in season or to suit your own taste.

1 cup/125g fresh or thawed frozen raspberries

1 cup/175g fresh or thawed frozen diced mango

4 tablespoons ground chia seeds

Optional garnishes: diced mango, fresh raspberries, sunflower seeds or pumpkin seeds

In a high-powered blender, combine the raspberries, mango, and ½ cup/120ml of water and blend until smooth. Pour the mixture into two dessert bowls or glass jars. Add 2 tablespoons of the ground chia seeds to each bowl and stir until evenly distributed. Cover and refrigerate for 8 hours or overnight. Serve as is or topped with garnish of choice.

IS MELAMINE SAFE?

Melamine, used to make inexpensive, hard plastic kitchenware, isn't suitable for microwaves and cooking,[98] but what about for just eating or drinking? Exposure to the chemical compound is significantly associated with kidney function deterioration in patients with early-stage chronic kidney disease,[99] so I'd skip melamine altogether.

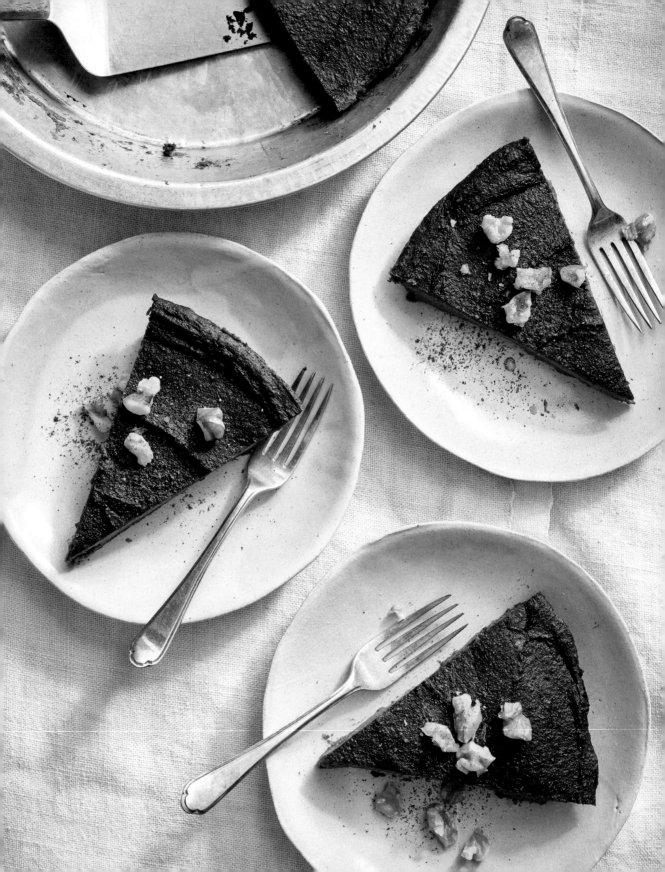

CRUST-FREE PUMPKIN PIE

MAKES: *6 to 8 servings*   DIFFICULTY: *Easy*

No need to feel deprived of a special dessert around the holidays with this pumpkin pie that is free of crust, sugar and dairy, but filled with the great taste of pumpkin and spices.

3 tablespoons ground chia seeds

1 cup/150g raw unsalted cashews, soaked in hot water for 30 minutes and then drained

1 (400g) BPA-free tin solid-pack pumpkin puree (*not* pumpkin pie filling)

⅓ cup/115g treacle, at room temperature

⅓ cup/75ml Date Syrup (page 217), at room temperature

1 tablespoon pumpkin pie spice or mixed spice

1 teaspoon pure vanilla extract

TO SERVE

⅓ cup/40g chopped walnuts (optional)

Preheat the oven to 180°C/350°F/gas mark 4.

In a small bowl, combine the ground chia seeds and 3 tablespoons of water, stirring to mix well. Set aside for 10 minutes to thicken.

Combine the drained cashews and the chia mixture in a high-powered blender and blend until the nuts are finely ground. Add the pumpkin puree, treacle, Date Syrup, pumpkin pie or mixed spice and vanilla and blend until smooth and creamy, about 2 minutes, stopping to scrape down the sides as needed.

Transfer the mixture into a 9-inch/23cm pie plate and bake for 45 minutes, or until the top looks cooked. Let the pie cool completely to room temperature, 1 to 2 hours, and then refrigerate until chilled and firm, about 3 hours. Keep refrigerated for up to 3 days.

To serve, cut into wedges and garnish with chopped walnuts, if desired.

BLACK FOREST CHIA PUDDING

MAKES: *2 servings*   DIFFICULTY: *Easy*

This decadent-tasting pudding can be enjoyed as a dessert, breakfast or snack.

1½ cups/340g pitted fresh or thawed frozen cherries

½ cup/150g mashed ripe banana

3 tablespoons unsweetened cocoa powder

2 pitted soft dates, soaked for 10 minutes in hot water and then drained

2 tablespoons ground chia seeds

Optional garnishes: fresh pitted cherries or berries, slivered almonds, or cacao nibs

In a high-powered blender or food processor, combine the cherries, banana, cocoa, dates, and ½ cup/120ml of water. Blend until completely smooth and divide evenly into two dessert bowls or glass jars. Add 1 tablespoon of the ground chia seeds to each bowl and stir until they are evenly distributed.

Cover and refrigerate for 8 hours or overnight. Serve as is or topped with garnish of choice.

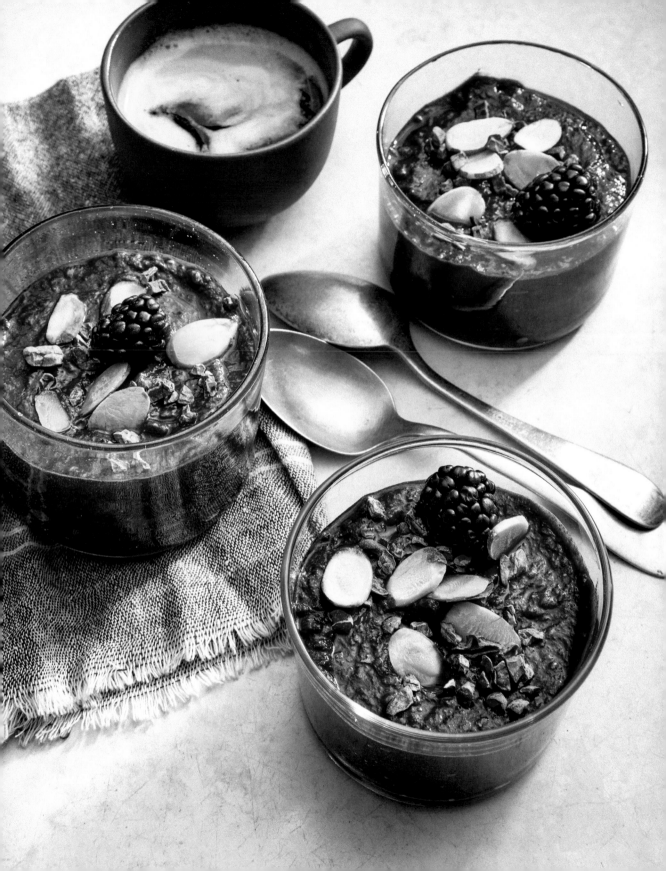

BAKED APPLES WITH WALNUTS AND GOJI BERRIES

MAKES: *4 servings*   DIFFICULTY: *Easy*

These luscious baked apples taste like apple pie, but aren't bogged down with added sugar, flour and fat. Another bonus is how great your house will smell while they're baking.

---

3 tablespoons goji berries, soaked in warm water for 15 minutes and then drained

⅓ cup/40g chopped walnuts

1 tablespoon Date Syrup (page 217)

1½ teaspoons ground cinnamon

4 large, firm baking apples, washed and cored

1 tablespoon fresh lemon juice

Preheat the oven to 180°C/350°F/gas mark 4.

Place the goji berries in a food processor and add the walnuts, Date Syrup and cinnamon; then pulse until well mixed. Set aside.

Peel the top third of each apple. Rub the exposed part of the apples with the lemon juice to prevent discoloration. Stuff about 2 tablespoons of the goji mixture into the centre of each apple and arrange the apples upright in a small, shallow baking dish. Pour ½ cup/120ml of water around the apples. Cover and bake until tender, about 1 hour. Serve warm.

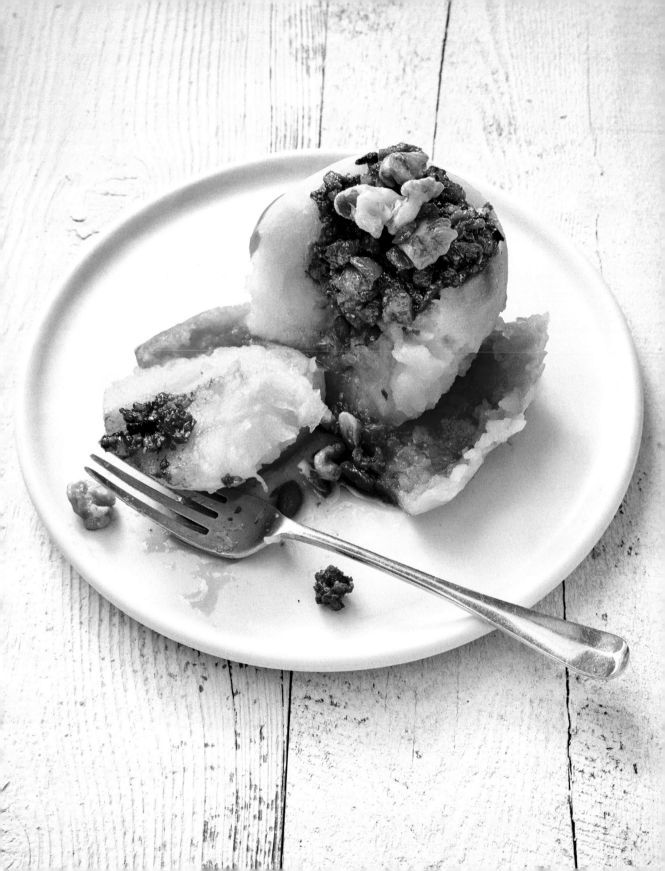

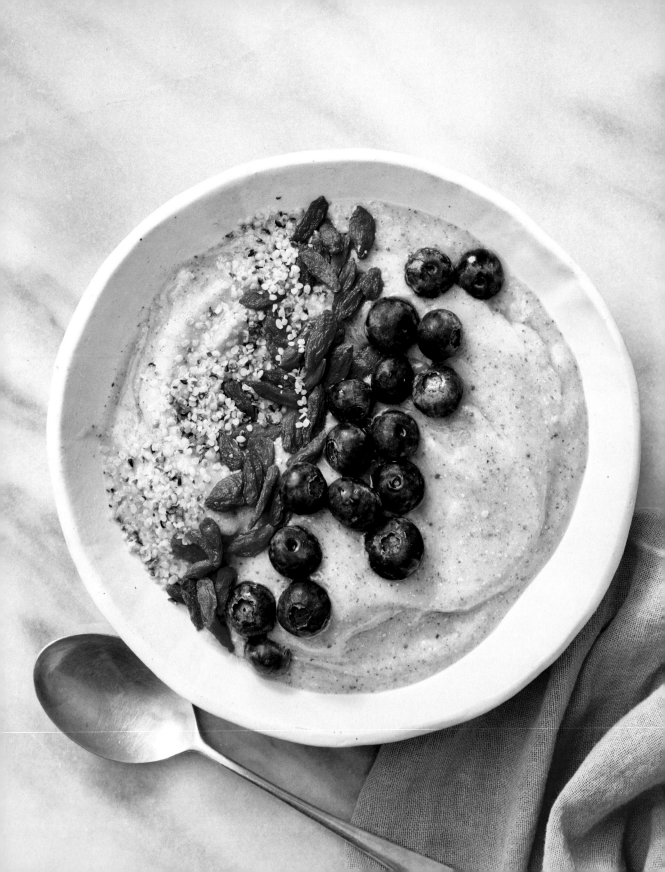

TROPICAL SMOOTHIE BOWLS

MAKES: *2 servings*   DIFFICULTY: *Easy*

Satisfying, delicious and versatile, smoothie bowls are thick smoothies you can eat with a spoon. This is the ultimate customizable dish: change up the fruits to suit your own taste and use whichever toppings you prefer. Smoothie bowls are especially good for breakfast or dessert. I like to keep banana chunks in my freezer so I always have them on hand. Frozen mango and pineapple, readily available in supermarkets, are convenient and often less expensive than fresh.

2 tablespoons ground chia seeds

2 ripe bananas, peeled, cut into chunks and frozen

1 cup/175g diced fresh or frozen mango

1 cup/200g diced fresh or frozen pineapple

Optional toppings: goji berries, sliced banana, berries, cacao nibs, ground flaxseeds or hemp seeds

Combine the ground chia seeds and ½ cup/120ml of water in a bowl and set aside for 10 minutes to thicken.

In a blender, combine the bananas, mango and pineapple. Add the chia seed mixture and blend until smooth.

Divide the smoothie mixture between two bowls. Add any desired toppings and serve.

GINGER ROASTED PEARS

MAKES: *2 to 4 servings*   DIFFICULTY: *Easy*

Roasted pears are easy to prepare and a lovely finish to a meal. For an extra flourish, garnish with a sprinkling of cacao nibs or crushed pistachios.

2 large ripe pears

1 tablespoon Date Syrup (page 217)

1 tablespoon fresh lemon juice

1 teaspoon ground ginger

Preheat the oven to 180°C/350°F/gas mark 4.

Cut the pears in half lengthways. Use a melon baller or a measuring spoon to scoop out the seeds. Place the pear halves, cut side up, on a rimmed baking tray.

In a small bowl, combine the Date Syrup and lemon juice and mix until well combined. (You may want to microwave the Date Syrup and lemon juice for 10 to 15 seconds so they blend more easily.)

Rub the cut side of each pear with the date mixture, then sprinkle with the ground ginger. Roast the pears in the oven for 30 minutes, or until just tender. Remove from the oven and allow to cool slightly before serving.

GROUND GINGER AND MUSCLE PAIN

Does ginger help with muscle pain? Apparently not acutely, so you can't just take it as you would a drug, but it may attenuate the day-to-day progression of muscle pain.[100] A teaspoon or two for a couple of days or weeks may reduce muscle pain and soreness as well as accelerate recovery of muscular strength.[101]

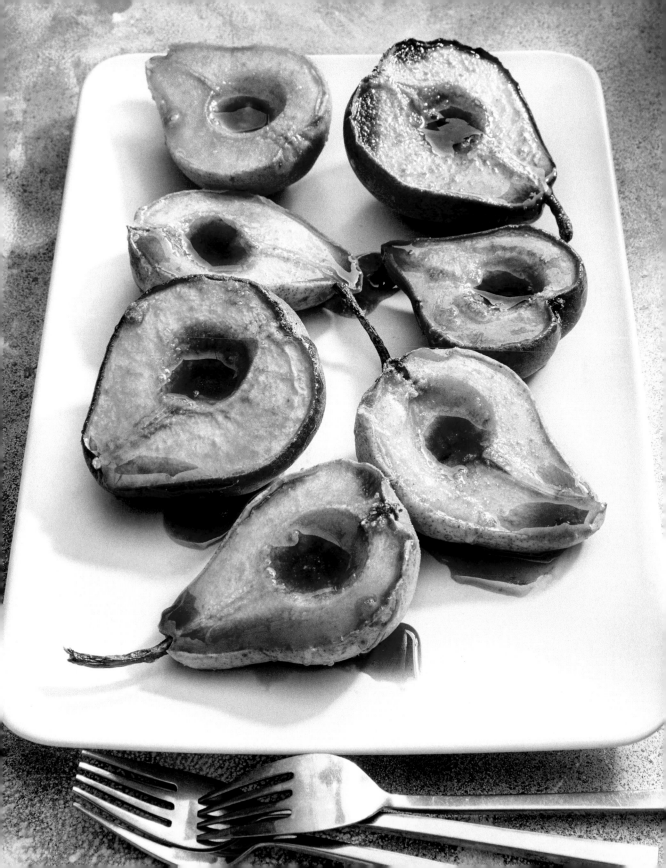

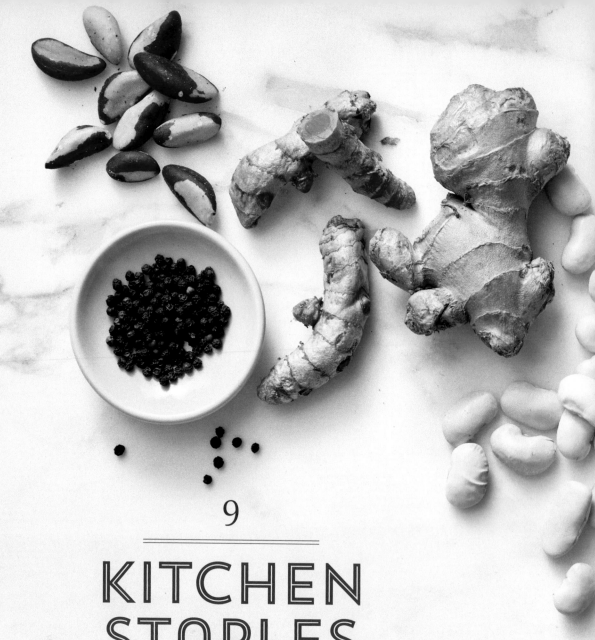

9

KITCHEN STAPLES

The recipes in this collection are for some of my must-have, go-to, make-everything-better sauces and spices, and bases and broths. At any given time, I have these in my pantry and refrigerator so they're on hand whenever I need them. I hope they become some of your favourites, too.

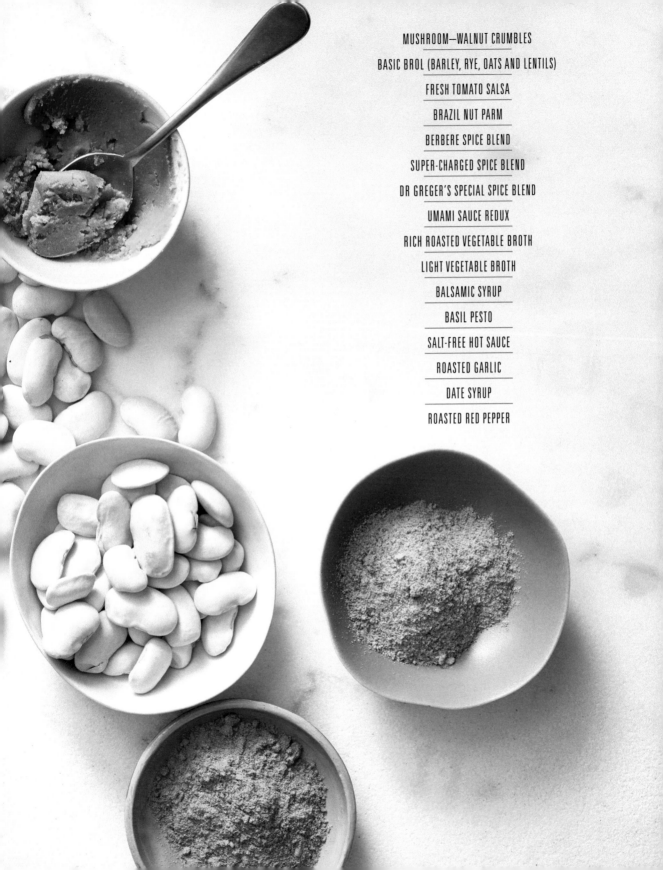

MUSHROOM—WALNUT CRUMBLES

BASIC BROL (BARLEY, RYE, OATS AND LENTILS)

FRESH TOMATO SALSA

BRAZIL NUT PARM

BERBERE SPICE BLEND

SUPER-CHARGED SPICE BLEND

DR GREGER'S SPECIAL SPICE BLEND

UMAMI SAUCE REDUX

RICH ROASTED VEGETABLE BROTH

LIGHT VEGETABLE BROTH

BALSAMIC SYRUP

BASIL PESTO

SALT-FREE HOT SAUCE

ROASTED GARLIC

DATE SYRUP

ROASTED RED PEPPER

MUSHROOM–WALNUT CRUMBLES

MAKES: *2 cups/250g*   DIFFICULTY: *Easy*

These crumbles add tremendous texture and flavour. Sprinkle them on top of cooked whole grains and vegetables, or add them to stuffing and pasta. The savoury flavour is similar to Italian sausage. For a spicy kick, add ½ teaspoon of red pepper flakes and use the optional cayenne.

6 ounces/175g baby portobello mushrooms
½ cup/60g walnut pieces
⅓ cup/45g raw sunflower seeds
⅓ cup/45g raw pumpkin seeds
¼ cup/30g ground flaxseeds
3 tablespoons nutritional yeast
1 teaspoon smoked paprika
1 teaspoon onion powder
1 teaspoon garlic powder
1 teaspoon ground fennel seeds
1 teaspoon dried oregano
1 teaspoon dried basil
¼ teaspoon cayenne (optional)
¼ teaspoon ground black pepper

Pulse the mushrooms in a food processor until finely chopped. Transfer to a bowl and set aside.

In the same food processor (no need to wipe it out), combine the walnuts, sunflower seeds and pumpkin seeds and pulse to coarsely grind. Add the ground nuts and seeds to the bowl of finely chopped mushrooms. Add all the remaining ingredients. Mix well.

Heat a large skillet or heavy-based frying pan over a medium heat. Cook the mixture, stirring frequently, for 10 minutes, or until the mushroom liquid has been released and evaporated, and crumbles begin to form. Cook a few minutes longer, until the crumbles begin to crisp. Remove from the heat and allow to cool. Use the crumbles immediately in recipes, or store them in an airtight container in the refrigerator for up to 3 days or in the freezer for up to 1 month.

For Variation: Substitute cold cooked whole grains (barley is a good choice) or grated cauliflower for the mushrooms.

BASIC BROL (BARLEY, RYE, OATS AND LENTILS)

MAKES: *5 cups/900g*   **DIFFICULTY:** *Easy*

BROL stands for barley, rye, oats and lentils. Barley groats, sold as pot or hull-less barley, rye grains, and oat groats are available in well-stocked supermarkets or online. Use purple barley, if you can find it, for the extra antioxidant boost. For the same reason, I use black lentils because they are the most antioxidant-packed lentils. Sometimes sold as beluga lentils due to their resemblance to caviar, you can also find black lentils in well-stocked supermarkets or online. For a gluten-free version of my Basic BROL, use gluten-free oats and substitute sorghum and millet for the rye and barley (SMOL!). Finger millet is one of the healthiest types. For convenience, you may want to cook your whole grains and lentils in larger proportions, then portion and freeze them for future use.

½ cup/100g dried black lentils, rinsed

½ cup/100g pot barley, rinsed

½ cup/85g rye grains, rinsed

½ cup/90g oat groats, rinsed

In an electric pressure cooker or multicooker, such as an Instant Pot, pressure-cook the lentils in 1 cup/250ml of water on high. (I use the Steam setting.) Allow time for natural pressure release so the remaining water gets absorbed. Remove the cooked lentils from the pot and set aside.

Combine the barley, rye and oat groats in the cooker. Stir in 3 cups/750ml of water. Pressure cook for 30 minutes, or use the Mixed Grain button if your cooker has one.

Add the cooked lentils to the cooked grains and toss gently to combine. The Basic BROL is now ready to use in recipes. You can also portion and freeze to use as needed.

For Variation: If you prefer to cook your whole grains on the stovetop, cook them separately, or cook them in larger amounts. Turn to the *Legumes and Grains Cooking Charts* on pages 218–221 for instruction, if needed.

FRESH TOMATO SALSA

MAKES: *3 cups/500g*   DIFFICULTY: *Easy*

Salsa is simple to make and especially delicious when fresh tomatoes are in season. Best of all, you can have it your way without the added salt and other ingredients often found in commercial salsas.

---

6 firm plum tomatoes, cored and coarsely chopped

½ pepper of any colour, de-seeded and finely chopped

2 tablespoons finely chopped red onion

1 jalapeño pepper or other small hot chilli, de-seeded and finely chopped

1 tablespoon apple cider vinegar

2 tablespoons finely chopped fresh coriander or parsley

Super-Charged Spice Blend (page 211)

Combine all the ingredients, including the Super-Charged Spice Blend to taste, in a bowl and stir to combine. Cover and let stand at room temperature for 1 hour before serving. If not using right away, store in an airtight container in the refrigerator. The salsa will keep refrigerated for 3 to 4 days.

BRAZIL NUT PARM

MAKES: *1½ cups/200g*   DIFFICULTY: *Easy*

I store this topping in a glass shaker with large holes and a tight-fitting lid so I can easily sprinkle it onto pasta and whole-grain dishes or salads for a cheesy flavour. Although the recipe calls for Brazil nuts and cashews, I sometimes mix it up and substitute other varieties of nuts. Experiment creatively and enjoy!

¾ cup/100g raw Brazil nuts

¼ cup/40g raw cashews

½ cup/70g nutritional yeast

2 teaspoons Dr Greger's Special Spice Blend (page 212)

Combine all the ingredients in a food processor and process until the nuts are finely ground. Transfer to a covered container or shaker with a tight-fitting lid and keep refrigerated. The Brazil Nut Parm will keep for up to 1 week in the refrigerator or 1 month in the freezer.

BERBERE SPICE BLEND

MAKES: *⅓ cup/100g*   DIFFICULTY: *Easy*

Because this spice blend features several spices, it's more economical to buy a small amount of the various spices sold in bulk, if available. You can also buy ready-made berbere in spice shops, ethnic markets or online.

3 tablespoons paprika

1 tablespoon cayenne, or to taste

2 teaspoons ground coriander

1 teaspoon ground ginger

1 teaspoon ground turmeric

1 teaspoon ground cumin

1 teaspoon onion powder

½ teaspoon ground cardamom

½ teaspoon ground fenugreek seeds

½ teaspoon ground black pepper

¼ teaspoon ground nutmeg

⅛ teaspoon ground cloves

⅛ teaspoon ground cinnamon

⅛ teaspoon ground allspice

Combine all the ingredients in a spice grinder or small food processor and grind finely to mix well. Transfer the spice mixture to a small jar with a tight-fitting lid and store in a cool, dry place.

SUPER-CHARGED SPICE BLEND

MAKES: *⅔ cup/50g*   DIFFICULTY: *Easy*

Similar to Dr Greger's Special Spice Blend from *The How Not to Die Cookbook*, included in this collection on page 212, this super-charged spice blend boasts the added benefits of cumin, nigella seeds, ginger and black pepper. I always have this seasoning blend on hand to boost flavours or to use in place of salt.

¼ cup/35g nutritional yeast

1 tablespoon garlic powder

1 tablespoon onion powder

1 tablespoon dried parsley

1 tablespoon dried basil

2 teaspoons ground thyme

2 teaspoons mustard powder

2 teaspoons paprika

2 teaspoons ground cumin

1 teaspoon ground nigella seeds

1 teaspoon ground ginger

½ teaspoon ground turmeric

½ teaspoon celery seeds

½ teaspoon ground black pepper

Combine all the ingredients in a spice grinder to mix well and pulverize the dried herbs. Transfer the mixture to a shaker bottle with a tight-fitting lid. Store in a cool, dry place.

DR GREGER'S SPECIAL SPICE BLEND

MAKES: *½ cup/120g* DIFFICULTY: *Easy*

For those times when your food needs seasoning without the flavour of cumin, here's my original spice blend recipe from *The How Not to Die Cookbook*.

2 tablespoons nutritional yeast

1 tablespoon onion powder

1 tablespoon dried parsley

1 tablespoon dried basil

2 teaspoons ground thyme

2 teaspoons garlic powder

2 teaspoons mustard powder

2 teaspoons paprika

½ teaspoon ground turmeric

½ teaspoon celery seeds

Combine all the ingredients in a spice grinder to mix well and pulverize the dried herbs. Transfer the mixture to a shaker bottle with a tight-fitting lid. Store in a cool, dry place.

UMAMI SAUCE REDUX

MAKES: *1¼ cups/300ml* DIFFICULTY: *Easy*

Umami is one of the five basic tastes, though many people are only learning about it now. The word was created by a Japanese chemist named Kikunae Ikeda from *umai*, which means 'delicious', and *mi*, which means 'taste'. This new and improved umami sauce is perfect in sautés or stir-fries to boost flavour without adding the sodium of salt or soy sauce.

1 cup/250ml Light Vegetable Broth (page 214)

1 teaspoon finely chopped garlic

1 teaspoon grated ginger

1½ tablespoons treacle

1 teaspoon salt-free tomato puree

½ teaspoon ground black pepper

2 teaspoons miso paste blended into 2 tablespoons water

1 tablespoon apple cider vinegar

1 tablespoon fresh lemon juice

Heat the Light Vegetable Broth in a small saucepan over a medium heat. Add the garlic and ginger and simmer for 3 minutes. Stir in the treacle, tomato puree and black pepper, and bring just to the boil.

Lower the heat to low and simmer for 1 minute. Remove from the heat, and then stir in the miso mixture, apple cider vinegar and lemon juice. Blend well. Taste and adjust the seasonings, if needed. Allow the sauce to cool before transferring to a jar or bottle with a tight-fitting lid. The sauce will keep in the refrigerator for up to 1 week. Alternatively, pour the cooled sauce into an ice cube tray and freeze into individual portions.

RICH ROASTED VEGETABLE BROTH

MAKES: *6-8 cups/1.5-2 litres*   DIFFICULTY: *Easy*

Use this broth in any recipes when you want to enrich the flavour of the dish. For a lighter broth, use the Light Vegetable Broth on page 214.

---

1 large onion, cut into wedges

1 red pepper, de-seeded and cut into 2-inch/5cm pieces

2 celery stalks, cut into 2-inch/5cm pieces

2 to 3 carrots, cut into 2-inch/5cm pieces

2 garlic cloves, coarsely chopped

8 ounces/225g baby portobello mushrooms, quartered

8 ounces/225g tomatoes, cored and halved

3 tablespoons white miso paste

2 tablespoons salt-free tomato puree

1 bunch parsley, chopped

1 bay leaf

6 whole black peppercorns

1 strip kombu (dried sea vegetable) (optional)

Preheat the oven to 220°C/425°F/gas mark 7. Line a large roasting tin or rimmed baking tray with a silicone mat or baking parchment. (You may need to use two trays.)

Spread the vegetables evenly in the prepared tin.

Roast the vegetables in the oven, stirring occasionally, until lightly browned and slightly caramelized, about 60 minutes. Remove the tin from the oven and transfer the roasted vegetables to a large soup pot. Stir in the miso paste and tomato puree. Add the parsley, bay leaf, peppercorns, kombu (if using) and 2.85 litres of water. Bring to the boil, then lower the heat to a simmer. Cook, uncovered, until the liquid is reduced by about half. Remove from the heat and allow to cool. Pour the broth through a colander into a large bowl or pot. The Rich Roasted Vegetable Broth is now ready to use.

To store the broth, allow it to cool completely before portioning it into containers with tight-fitting lids. Refrigerate or freeze until needed.

Instead of discarding the vegetable solids, you can either eat them as is or, after removing and discarding the bay leaf, kombu and peppercorns, puree the vegetables and then portion and freeze them in small containers for later use to enrich soups or gravies.

For an even richer broth, add some of the pureed vegetables back into the broth before using.

LIGHT VEGETABLE BROTH

MAKES: *6 cups/1.5 litres*   **DIFFICULTY:** *Easy*

Use this light, all-purpose salt-free broth in any recipe calling for any kind of broth.

1 red onion, coarsely chopped

2 carrots, cut into 1-inch/2.5cm pieces

2 celery stalks, coarsely chopped

3 garlic cloves, crushed

2 plum tomatoes, cored and halved

2 dried shiitake mushrooms

1 (2-inch/5cm) piece of kombu (dried sea vegetable) (optional)

½ cup/15g fresh, coarsely chopped parsley

2 bay leaves

½ teaspoon ground black pepper

2 tablespoons white miso paste

Dr Greger's Special Spice Blend (page 212)

In a large pot, heat 1 cup/250ml of water over a medium heat. Add the onion, carrot, celery and garlic and cook for 5 minutes. Stir in the tomatoes, mushrooms, kombu (if using), parsley, bay leaves and black pepper. Add 7 cups/1.75 litres of water and bring to the boil. Lower the heat to low and simmer for 1½ hours.

Remove from the heat, let cool slightly; then remove and discard the kombu if used. Transfer the broth to a high-powered blender and blend until smooth. Strain the blended broth through a fine-mesh sieve back into the pot or a large bowl, pressing the vegetables against the sieve to release their juices. Ladle about ⅓ cup/75ml of the broth into a small bowl or cup. Add the miso paste and Dr Greger's Special Spice Blend to taste and stir well before incorporating back into the broth.

Let the broth cool to room temperature before dividing into containers with tight-sealing lids and storing in the refrigerator or freezer. Properly stored, the broth will keep for up to 5 days in the refrigerator or up to 3 months in the freezer.

COOKING TO LIVE LONGER

Food prepared at home tends to have less saturated fat, cholesterol and sodium, and more fibre,[102] so benefits may include chronic disease prevention.[103] But do people who cook live longer? Yes! Those who cooked more than five times a week versus not at all had higher vegetable consumption[104] and only 59 per cent of the mortality risk. So, put on that apron!

BALSAMIC SYRUP

MAKES: *½ cup/120ml*   **DIFFICULTY:** *Easy*

Three tips for you: First, be sure to watch carefully when reducing the vinegar so it doesn't reduce too much and burn. Second, if the syrup hardens after being refrigerated, place the container in a bowl filled with warm water to gently warm it. And, third, double, triple or make even more of the recipe, depending on how much you want to have on hand.

---

1 cup/250ml balsamic vinegar

Pour the vinegar into a small saucepan and bring just to the boil. Lower the heat to a low simmer and allow the vinegar to reduce by about half, or until it is thick enough to coat the back of a spoon. Watch closely so it doesn't burn. The reduction should take 15 to 20 minutes (or longer if you make a larger quantity). Remove from the heat and allow to cool. The syrup will continue to thicken as it cools. Once cool, it is ready to use. If not using right away, transfer the syrup to an airtight container and store at room temperature or in the refrigerator. It keeps for up to 3 days at room temperature or 2 weeks in the fridge.

BASIL PESTO

MAKES: *2 cups/200g*   **DIFFICULTY:** *Easy*

For convenience, portion this pesto and freeze it for future use. (A silicone ice cube tray works well for this.)

---

3 garlic cloves, crushed

½ cup/75g raw unsalted cashews, soaked for 30 minutes in hot water and then drained

⅓ cup/45g nutritional yeast

½ cup/60g walnut pieces

2 teaspoons white miso paste

3 cups/120g packed fresh basil leaves

1 teaspoon Dr Greger's Special Spice Blend (page 212), or to taste

In a food processor, combine the garlic, cashews, nutritional yeast and walnuts and process to a paste. Add the miso paste, basil, Dr Greger's Special Spice Blend and ¼ cup/60ml of water and process until smooth and combined. The Basil Pesto will stay fresh for 1 or 2 days in an airtight container in the refrigerator or up to 1 month in the freezer.

SALT-FREE HOT SAUCE

MAKES: *2 cups/500ml* **DIFFICULTY:** *Easy*

For the spice and heat without the salt found in most bottled hot sauces, look no further than this recipe. The type of chillies you use will determine the heat level of the sauce, but regardless of which hot chillies you use, be sure to use rubber gloves when handling them and do not touch your eyes.

---

12 ounces/350g fresh hot chillies of your choice, de-stemmed, halved lengthways, de-seeded and chopped

½ cup/75g chopped red onion

1 tablespoon finely chopped garlic

½–1 cup/120–250ml apple cider vinegar, to taste

In a saucepan, combine the chillies, onion, garlic and ¼ cup/60ml of water. Cook over a high heat, stirring, for 2 to 3 minutes. Lower the heat to medium-high, add 1¾ cups/425ml of water, and continue to cook, stirring occasionally, for 15 to 20 minutes, or until the chillies are very soft and the water is reduced by about half. Remove from the heat and let the mixture cool to room temperature.

Transfer the cooled mixture to a food processor and process until very smooth. Add ½ cup/120ml of the apple cider vinegar and process to blend. Taste the sauce and add more of the vinegar, if desired, according to your taste. Transfer the hot sauce into a clean glass jar or bottle, secure with an airtight lid, and keep refrigerated.

ROASTED GARLIC

MAKES: *3 tablespoons* **DIFFICULTY:** *Easy*

Roasted garlic is easy to make and can be used to add flavour to many of the recipes in this book.

---

1 whole head garlic

Preheat the oven to 200°C/400°F/gas mark 6.

Use a sharp knife to cut about ⅓ inch/1cm off the top of the garlic head to expose the tops of the garlic cloves. Place the bulb, cut side up, inside a terracotta garlic baker or wrap it securely in aluminium foil. Bake for 30 to 40 minutes, or until the garlic cloves are soft. Remove from the oven and open the garlic baker or foil to let the garlic cool. Remove one garlic clove and squeeze it over a small bowl, allowing the soft roasted garlic to slip out of the papery skin. If it is not very soft and golden brown, then return the rest of the bulb back to the garlic baker or rewrap it in the foil and bake for a few minutes longer. When the garlic is soft inside and cool enough to handle, squeeze the roasted garlic out of each clove and into the bowl. The Roasted Garlic is now ready to use and can be stored in the refrigerator in a jar or other container with a tight-fitting lid for up to 5 days.

GARLIC FOR CANCER AND THE COMMON COLD

Garlic lowers blood pressure, regulates cholesterol, stimulates immunity,[105] and may prevent occurrences of the common cold.[106] Is it also a stake through the heart of cancer?[107] Those who eat more garlic appear to have lower cancer rates than those who eat less.[108]

DATE SYRUP

MAKES: *1½ cups/370ml*   DIFFICULTY: *Easy*

Date Syrup is great to have on hand when you need a whole food sweetener.

---

1 cup/225g pitted dates

1 cup/250ml boiling water

1 teaspoon fresh lemon juice

Combine the dates and water in a heatproof bowl, and set aside for 1 hour to allow the dates to soften. Transfer the dates and the soaking water to a high-powered blender. Add the lemon juice and process until smooth. Transfer to a glass jar or other container with a tight-fitting lid. Store the syrup in the refrigerator for 2 to 3 weeks.

WHAT ABOUT STAINLESS-STEEL AND CAST-IRON COOKWARE?

Under day-to-day conditions, stainless-steel cook-ware is considered safe even for most people acutely sensitive to nickel and chromium,[109] and cast iron can help to improve iron status and potentially reduce anaemia incidence among reproductive-age women[110] and children.[111]

ROASTED RED PEPPER

MAKES: *1 pepper*   DIFFICULTY: *Easy*

Roasted red peppers add a beautiful colour and delicious smoky flavour to dishes. You can buy them water-packed in jars, but they're easy to make at home in the oven or on the stovetop – and homemade always tastes *so* much better!

---

1 large red pepper

IN THE OVEN: Set the oven to grill and place the pepper 8 inches/20cm from the heat source. Grill, turning every few minutes as needed, for about 15 minutes, or until much of the skin has blistered.

ON THE STOVETOP: Over high heat, cook the pepper either directly over an open flame or in a cast-iron skillet or griddle pan, turning every minute or so as needed with kitchen tongs, until it's mostly blistered.

Once the pepper is roasted, transfer it to a bowl. Cover tightly for about 15 minutes to allow the pepper to steam. (The heat from the pepper enables it to essentially steam itself, softening it and making it easier to remove the skin.)

After the pepper has steamed, remove it from the bowl and place it on a clean surface. Rub off the charred skin from the pepper (it should come off easily); then remove the stem with a paring knife and scrape out the seeds with a spoon. The Roasted Red Pepper is now ready to use in recipes.

COOKING CHARTS: LEGUMES AND GRAINS

Cooking legumes and whole grains is fairly formulaic. It's a simple process that results in amazingly delicious – and healthy – food. The following are instructions for preparing these staples on the stovetop or in a multicooker, such as an Instant Pot, or a pressure cooker.

COOKING LEGUMES ON THE STOVETOP

Generally, 1 cup of dried legumes yields about 3 cups of cooked legumes.

When cooking on a stovetop, dried legumes – with the exception of lentils – require soaking prior to cooking. Soaking rehydrates the legumes and shortens their cooking time. It also dissolves some of the complex sugars that cause digestive gas. Before soaking legumes, rinse them, and then pick through to remove any small stones or other debris.

To soak the legumes, place them in a bowl with enough water to cover them by about 3 inches (7.5cm). Soak them overnight and drain before cooking. To quick-soak legumes, put them in a pot with enough water to cover by about 3 inches (7.5cm) and boil for 2 minutes. Remove the pot from the heat, cover, and leave to stand for 2 hours before draining. The quick-soaked legumes are then ready for cooking.

STOVETOP COOKING TIMES FOR SOAKED LEGUMES

LEGUME (1 CUP DRIED)	WATER	COOKING TIME
Adzuki beans	3 cups	45 to 50 minutes
Black beans	4 cups	50 to 60 minutes
Black-eyed beans	3 cups	45 minutes
Cannellini beans (white)	4 cups	60 minutes
Chickpeas	4 cups	60 to 70 minutes
Great northern beans (white)	3½ cups	50 minutes
Kidney beans	3½ cups	50 to 60 minutes
Lentils (brown)* Lentils (black or green)* Lentils (red)*	3 cups 3 cups 3 cups	25 to 30 minutes 30 minutes 10 to 15 minutes
Navy beans	3½ cups	50 minutes
Pinto beans	3½ cups	50 minutes

*Note: Lentils do not require soaking.

Cooking time may vary, depending on the type, quality and age of the legumes as well as the altitude at which you are cooking. Cooked legumes should be firm but tender. Once cooked, drain in a colander and rinse with cold water before using.

Cooked legumes will keep well in an airtight container in the refrigerator for up to 5 days or in the freezer for 3 months or longer.

COOKING LEGUMES IN A MULTICOOKER OR PRESSURE COOKER

If you have a large (5.7–7.6 litres) multicooker, such as an Instant Pot, or another pressure cooker, you can cook 1 pound/450g (2 cups) of legumes at a time. Generally, 1 cup of dried legumes yields about 3 cups cooked.

Cooking time may vary, depending on the type, quality and age of the legumes as well as the altitude of your kitchen and variables among different appliances.

Rinse the dried legumes; then pick through to remove any small stones or other debris. Add the legumes to your cooker along with the water quantity specified in the following chart.

Close and lock the lid. Set the valve on the lid to Sealing. Select the Pressure Cook function with High Pressure. Cook on high pressure for the directed time. Let the pressure release naturally for at least 20 minutes.

Remove the lid. The legumes should be firm but tender. Once cooked, drain in a colander and rinse with cold water before using.

Cooked legumes will keep well in an airtight container in the refrigerator for up to 5 days or in the freezer for 3 months or longer.

MULTICOOKER COOKING TIMES FOR UNSOAKED LEGUMES ON HIGH PRESSURE

LEGUME (1 CUP DRIED)	WATER	COOKING TIME
Adzuki beans	2 cups	20 minutes
Black beans	3 cups	25 minutes
Black-eyed beans	3 cups	20 minutes
Cannellini beans (white)	4 cups	40 minutes
Chickpeas	4 cups	45 minutes
Great northern beans (white)	3 cups	35 minutes
Kidney beans	3 cups	30 minutes
Lentils (brown) Lentils (black or green) Lentils (red)	2 cups 2 cups 1¾ cups	8 minutes 8 minutes 5 minutes
Navy beans	3 cups	25 minutes
Pinto beans	3 cups	25 minutes

PRESSURE STEAMING GREENS?

I pour a layer of water into the bottom of my electric pressure cooker pot, drop in a metal steamer basket, add greens, and steam them under pressure. The small feet on metal steamer baskets keep the water from touching the food, and you can get the same delicious, melt-in-your-mouth texture of traditional southern collards and Ethiopian greens by just steaming under pressure for one minute or less. Release the steam, and the greens are perfect – bright emerald green and cooked tender.

NOTE: There is no need to soak legumes when cooking them in a multicooker or pressure cooker. They will cook well without the overnight soak or quick-soak needed for stovetop cooking. However, some people find that soaking legumes helps make them easier to digest. If you choose to presoak before pressure-cooking, be aware that the cooking time for presoaked legumes in the cooker will be reduced significantly. Generally, presoaking will cut the cooking time in half or even more.

COOKING WHOLE GRAINS ON THE STOVETOP

Generally, 1 cup of uncooked whole grains yields about 3 cups of cooked whole grains.

Before you cook any grains, be sure to rinse them to remove loose hulls, dust, and other impurities. Longer-cooking grains, such as rye grains and oat groats, should be soaked overnight and then drained.

To cook grains, add them to a pot and cover with 2 to 3 times as much water. (Adding extra water for longer-cooking grains will help keep them from scorching, and any excess water can be drained off.) Bring the water to the boil, then lower the heat to low, cover, and simmer for the average time specified in the following chart until tender.

If the grains are not tender before the water is absorbed, add a little more water and continue to cook until the grains are to your liking. After cooking, remove the pot from the heat and let it stand, covered, for 5 to 10 minutes before serving. If any water remains in the pot, drain it off before serving. When ready to serve, fluff the grains with a fork.

Cooked grains will keep well in an airtight container in the refrigerator for up to 5 days or in the freezer for 3 months or longer.

STOVETOP COOKING TIMES FOR WHOLE GRAINS

GRAIN (1 CUP DRIED)	WATER	COOKING TIME
Barley (pot)	3 to 4 cups	50 to 60 minutes
Millet	2½ cups	30 minutes
Oat groats	3 to 4 cups	50 to 60 minutes
Quinoa	2 cups	15 to 20 minutes
Rye grains	3 to 4 cups	60 minutes
Sorghum	3 to 4 cups	50 to 60 minutes
Teff	2 cups	15 to 20 minutes

COOKING WHOLE GRAINS IN A MULTICOOKER OR PRESSURE COOKER

Generally, 1 cup of uncooked whole grains yields about 3 cups of cooked whole grains. If you have a large (6- to 8-quart) multicooker, such as an Instant Pot, or another pressure cooker, you can cook 2 cups of grains at a time.

Before you cook any grains, rinse them to remove loose hulls, dust, and other impurities. There is no need to soak any grains when cooking in an Instant Pot.

Add the grains and the water quantity specified in the following chart to your multicooker or pressure cooker. Close and lock the lid. Set the valve on the lid to Sealing. Select the Pressure Cook function with High Pressure. Cook on high pressure for the directed time. Let the pressure release naturally for at least 20 minutes.

Remove the lid. The grains should be firm but tender. If any water remains, drain the grains in a colander. When ready to serve, fluff the grains with a fork.

Cooked grains will keep well in an airtight container in the refrigerator for up to 5 days or in the freezer for 3 months or longer.

DOES PRESSURE COOKING PRESERVE NUTRIENTS?

Pressure cooking presoaked black beans for 15 minutes, for example, results in six times more antioxidant content than boiling for an hour,[112] and pressure cooking carrots nearly doubles antioxidant value. There was significantly less nutrient loss when pressure cooking spinach for three and a half minutes compared to boiling for eight.[113]

MULTICOOKER COOKING TIMES FOR WHOLE GRAINS ON HIGH PRESSURE

GRAIN (1 CUP DRIED)	WATER	COOKING TIME
Barley (pot)	3 cups	20 to 30 minutes
Millet	2 cups	8 to 10 minutes
Oat groats	3 cups	20 to 30 minutes
Quinoa	2 cups	1 minute
Rye grain	3 cups	20 to 30 minutes
Sorghum	3 cups	20 to 30 minutes
Teff	2 cups	2 to 3 minutes

REFERENCES

1 J. M. Westfall, J. Mold, and L. Fagnan, '"Blue Highways" on the NIH Roadmap', *JAMA* 297, no. 4 (2007): 403–06.

2 D. Ornish, S. E. Brown, L. W. Scherwitz, et al., 'Can Lifestyle Changes Reverse Coronary Heart Disease? The Lifestyle Heart Trial', *Lancet* 336, no. 8708 (1990): 129–33.

3 J. Allen, D. R. Anderson, B. Baun, et al., 'Reflections on Developments in Health Promotion in the Past Quarter Century from Founding Members of the *American Journal of Health Promotion* Editorial Board', *Am J Health Promot* 25, no. 4 (2011): ei–eviii.

4 K. Casazza, K. R. Fontaine, A. Astrup, et al., 'Myths, Presumptions, and Facts about Obesity', *N Engl J Med* 368, no. 5 (2013): 446–54.

5 N. Wright, L. Wilson, M. Smith, B. Duncan, and P. Mchugh, 'The BROAD Study: A Randomised Controlled Trial Using a Whole Food Plant-Based Diet in the Community for Obesity, Ischaemic Heart Disease or Diabetes', *Nutr Diabetes* 7, no. 3 (2017): e256.

6 C. B. Esselstyn, 'A Plant-Based Diet and Coronary Artery Disease: A Mandate for Effective Therapy', *J Geriatr Cardiol* 14, no. 5 (2017): 317–20.

7 J. W. Anderson and K. Ward, 'High-Carbohydrate, High-Fiber Diets for Insulin-Treated Men with Diabetes Mellitus', *Am J Clin Nutr* 32, no. 11 (1979): 2312–21.

8 R. K. Calder and A. J. Mussap, 'Factors Influencing Women's Choice of Weight-Loss Diet', *J Health Psychol* 20, no. 5 (2015): 612–24.

9 S. Ramage, A. Farmer, K. A. Eccles, and I. McCargar, 'Healthy Strategies for Successful Weight Loss and Weight Maintenance: A Systematic Review', *Appl Physiol Nutr Metab* 39, no. 1 (2014): 1–20.

10 W. C. Willett, 'The Dietary Pyramid: Does The Foundation Need Repair?' *Am J Clin Nutr* 68, no. 2 (1998): 218–19.

11 C. J. Rebello, C. E. O'Neil, and F. L. Greenway, 'Dietary Fiber and Satiety: The Effects of Oats on Satiety', *Nutr Rev* 74, no. 2 (2016): 131–47.

12 E. A. Decker, D. J. Rose, and D. Stewart, 'Processing of Oats and the Impact of Processing Operations on Nutrition and Health Benefits', *Br J Nutr* 112 Suppl. 2 (2014): S58–64.

13 Ibid.

14 H. Kahleova, A. Tura, M. Hill, R. Holubkov, and N. D. Barnard, 'A Plant-Based Dietary Intervention Improves Beta-Cell Function and Insulin Resistance in Overweight Adults: A 16-Week Randomized Clinical Trial', *Nutrients* 10, no. 2 (2018): 189.

15 J. Sabaté and M. Wien, 'Vegetarian Diets and Childhood Obesity Prevention', *Am J Clin Nutr* 91, no. 5 (2010): 1525S–29S.

16 E. Guth, 'Healthy Weight Loss', *JAMA* 312, no. 9 (2014): 974.

17 M. Greger, 'Dr. Greger in the Kitchen: My New Favorite Beverage', NutritionFacts.org, published November 13, 2017, available at https://nutritionfacts .org/video/dr-greger-in-the-kitchen-my-new-favorite-beverage, accessed April 17, 2019.

18 B. J. Rolls, E. A. Bell, and M. L. Thorwart, 'Water Incorporated into a Food but Not Served with a Food Decreases Energy Intake in Lean Women', *Am J Clin Nutr* 70, no. 4 (1999): 448–55.

19 A. Santangelo, M. Peracchi, D. Conte, M. Fraquelli, and M. Porrini, 'Physical State of Meal Affects Gastric Emptying, Cholecystokinin Release and Satiety', *Br J Nutr* 80, no. 6 (1998): 521–27.

20 Y. Zhu and J. H. Hollis, 'Soup Consumption Is Associated with a Lower Dietary Energy Density and a Better Diet Quality in US Adults', *Br J Nutr* 111, no. 8 (2014): 1474–80.

21 A. Lapointe, C. Couillard, and S. Lemieux, 'Effects of Dietary Factors on Oxidation of Low-Density Lipoprotein Particles', *J Nutr Biochem* 17, no. 10 (2006): 645–58.

22 T. Bacchetti, D. Tullii, S. Masciangelo, et al., 'Effect of Black and Red Cabbage on Plasma Carotenoid Levels, Lipid Profile and Oxidized Low Density Lipoprotein', *J Funct Foods* 8 (2014): 128–37.

23 M. Bouchenak and M. Lamri-Senhadji, 'Nutritional Quality of Legumes, and Their Role in Cardiometabolic Risk Prevention: A Review', *J Med Food* 16, no. 3 (2013): 185–98.

24 A. Drewnowski and C. D. Rehm, 'Vegetable Cost Metrics Show That Potatoes and Beans Provide Most Nutrients per Penny', *PLoS ONE* 8, no. 5 (2013): e63277.

25 M. Bouchenak and M. Lamri-Senhadji, 'Nutritional Quality of Legumes, and Their Role in Cardiometabolic Risk Prevention: A Review', *J Med Food* 16, no. 3 (2013): 185–98.

26 L. A. Bazzano, J. He, L. G. Ogden, et al., 'Legume Consumption and Risk of Coronary Heart Disease in US Men and Women: NHANES I Epidemiologic Follow-up Study', *Arch Intern Med* 161, no. 21 (2001): 2573–78.

Y. Abe, M. Mutsuga, H. Ohno, Y. Kawamura, and H. Akiyama, 'Isolation and Quantification of Polyamide Cyclic Oligomers in Kitchen Utensils and Their Migration into Various Food Simulants', *PLoS ONE* 11 (7) (2016;): e0159547.

27 Federal Institute for Risk Assessment, 'Polyamide Kitchen Utensils: Keep Contact with Hot Food as Brief as Possible', Federal Ministry of Food, Agriculture and Consumer Protection, BfR Opinion No. 036/2019, published September 17, 2019.

28 J. Kuang, M. A. Abdallah, and S. Harrad, 'Brominated Flame Retardants in Black Plastic Kitchen Utensils: Concentrations and Human Exposure Implications', *Sci Total Environ* 610–611 (2018): 1138–46.

29 S. M. Krebs-Smith, P. M. Guenther, A. F. Subar, S. I. Kirkpatrick, and K. W. Dodd, 'Americans Do Not Meet Federal Dietary Recommendations', *J Nutr* 140, no. 10 (2010): 1832–38.

30 D. C. Murador, D. T. da Cunha, and V. V. de Rosso, 'Effects of Cooking Techniques on Vegetable Pigments: A Meta-analytic Approach to Carotenoid and Anthocyanin Levels', *Food Res Int* 65 (pt. B) (2014): 177–83.

31 F. A. Ahmed and R. F. Ali, 'Bioactive Compounds and Antioxidant Activity of Fresh and Processed White Cauliflower', *Biomed Res Int* 2013 (2013): 367819.

32 A. Khor, R. Grant, C. Tung, et al., 'Postprandial Oxidative Stress Is Increased after a Phytonutrient-Poor Food but Not after a Kilojoule-Matched Phytonutrient-Rich Food', *Nutr Res* 34, no. 5 (2014): 391–400.

33 M. S. Islam, O. Protic, S. R. Giannubilo, et al., 'Uterine Leiomyoma: Available Medical Treatments and New Possible Therapeutic Options', *J Clin Endocrinol Metab* 98, no. 3 (2013): 921–34.

F. M. Steinberg, M. J. Murray, R. D. Lewis, et al., 'Clinical Outcomes of a 2-Y Soy Isoflavone Supplementation in Menopausal Women', *Am J Clin Nutr* 93, no. 2 (2011): 356–67.

34 L. S. McAnulty, S. R. Collier, M. J. Landram, et al., 'Six Weeks Daily Ingestion of Whole Blueberry Powder Increases Natural Killer Cell Counts and Reduces Arterial Stiffness in Sedentary Males and Females', *Nutr Res* 34, no. 7 (2014): 577–84.

35 S. Vendrame, S. Guglielmetti, P. Riso, S. Arioli, D. Klimis-Zacas, and M. Porrini, 'Six-Week Consumption of a Wild Blueberry Powder Drink Increases Bifidobacteria in the Human Gut', *J Agric Food Chem* 59, no. 24 (2011): 12815–20.

36 J. C. Kagan, 'Immunology: Sensing Endotoxins from Within', *Science* 341, no. 6151 (2013): 1184–85.

37 V. H. Tournas, 'Spoilage of Vegetable Crops by Bacteria and Fungi and Related Health Hazards', *Crit Rev Microbiol* 31, no. 1 (2005): 33–44.

38 S. Mishra and J. Monro, 'Wholeness and Primary and Secondary Food Structure Effects on *in Vitro* Digestion Patterns Determine Nutritionally Distinct Carbohydrate Fractions in Cereal Foods', *Food Chem* 135, no. 3 (2012): 1968–74.

39 B. Simonato, A. Curioni, and G. Pasini, 'Digestibility of Pasta Made with Three Wheat Types: A Preliminary Study', *Food Chem* 174, no. 2 (2015): 219–25.

40 G. Costabile, E. Griffo, P. Cipriano, et al., 'Subjective Satiety and Plasma PYY Concentration after Wholemeal Pasta', *Appetite* 125 (2018): 172–81.

41 M. Mahdavi-Roshan, P. Mirmiran, M. Arjmand, and J. Nasrollahzadeh, 'Effects of Garlic on Brachial Endothelial Function and Capacity of Plasma to Mediate Cholesterol Efflux in Patients with Coronary Artery Disease', *Anatol J Cardiol* 18, no. 2 (2017): 116–21.

42 N. Mahdavi-Roshan, A. Zahedmehr, A. Mohammad-Zadeh, et al., 'Effect of Garlic Powder Tablet on Carotid Intima-media Thickness in Patients with Coronary Artery Disease: A Preliminary Randomized Controlled Trial', *Nutr Health* 22, no. 2 (2013): 143–55.

43 X. J. Xiong, P. Q. Wang, S. J. Li, X. K. Li, Y. Q. Zhang, and J. Wang, 'Garlic for Hypertension: A Systematic Review and Meta-analysis of Randomized Controlled Trials', *Phytomedicine* 22, no. 3 (2015): 352–61.

44 P. Bowen, L. Chen, M. Stacewicz-Sapuntzakis, et al., 'Tomato Sauce Supplementation and Prostate Cancer: Lycopene Accumulation and Modulation of Biomarkers of Carcinogenesis', *Exp Biol Med (Maywood)* 227, no. 10 (2002): 886–93; L. Chen, M. Stacewicz-Sapuntzakis, C. Duncan, et al., 'Oxidative DNA Damage in Prostate Cancer Patients Consuming Tomato Sauce-Based Entrees as a Whole-Food Intervention,' *J Natl Cancer Inst* 93, no. 24 (2001): 1872–79.

45 R. P. Walsh, H. Bartlett, and F. Eperjesi, 'Variation in Carotenoid Content of Kale and Other Vegetables: A Review of Pre- and Post-harvest Effects', *J Agric Food Chem* 63, no. 44 (2015): 9677–82.

46 M. Greger, 'Prevent Glaucoma and See 27 Miles Farther', NutritionFacts.org, published May 18, 2012, available at https://nutritionfacts.org/video/prevent-glaucoma-and-see-27-miles-farther, accessed December 17, 2019.

47 M. Greger, 'Do Lutein Supplements Help with Brain Function?' NutritionFacts.org, published December 31, 2018, available at https://nutritionfacts.org/video/do-lutein-supplements-help-with-brain-function/, accessed December 17, 2019.

48 L. C. Dos Reis, V. R. de Oliveira, M. E. Hagen, A. Jablonski, S. H. Flôres, and A. de Oliveira Rios, 'Effect of Cooking on the Concentration of Bioactive Compounds in Broccoli (*Brassica oleracea var. Avenger)* and Cauliflower (*Brassica oleracea var. Alphina F1)* Grown in an Organic System', *Food Chem* 172 (2015): 770–77.

49 Ibid.

50 R. W. Welch, 'Satiety: Have We Neglected Dietary Non-nutrients?' *Proc Nutr Soc* 70, no. 2 (2011): 145–54.

51 E. Wisker and W. Feldheim, 'Metabolizable Energy of Diets Low or High in Dietary Fiber from Fruits and Vegetables When Consumed by Humans', *J Nutr* 120, no. 11 (1990): 1331–37.

52 L. Liu, S. Wang, and J. Liu, 'Fiber Consumption and All-Cause, Cardiovascular, and Cancer Mortalities: A Systematic Review and Meta-analysis of Cohort Studies', *Mol Nutr Food Res* 59, no. 1 (2015): 139–46.

53 A. Wald, 'Constipation: Advances in Diagnosis and Treatment', *JAMA* 315, no. 2 (2016): 214.

54 M. Petrie, W. J. Rejeski, S. Basu, et al., 'Beet Root Juice: An Ergogenic Aid for Exercise and the Aging Brain', *J Gerontol A Biol Sci Med Sci* 72, no. 9 (2017): 1284–89.

55 A. Cassidy, G. Rogers, J. J. Peterson, J. T. Dwyer, H. Lin, and P. F. Jacques, 'Higher Dietary Anthocyanin and Flavonol Intakes Are Associated with Anti-inflammatory Effects in a Population of US Adults', *Am J Clin Nutr* 102, no. 1 (2015): 172–81.

56 I. Edirisinghe, K. Banaszewski, J. Cappozzo, et al., 'Strawberry Anthocyanin and its Association with Postprandial Inflammation and Insulin', *Br J Nutr* 106, no. 6 (2011): 913–22.

57 US Department of Health and Human Services, US Department of Agriculture, 'Food Sources of Dietary Fiber', *2015–2020 Dietary Guidelines for Americans*, 8th ed., app. 13, DietaryGuidelines.gov, published December 2015, available at https://health.gov/dietaryguidelines/2015/guidelines/appendix-13, accessed March 31, 2019.

58 J. N. Davis, K. E. Alexander, E. E. Ventura, C. M. Toledo-Corral, and M. I. Goran, 'Inverse Relation Between Dietary Fiber Intake and Visceral Adiposity in Overweight Latino Youth', *Am J Clin Nutr* 90, no. 5 (2009): 1160–66.

59 L. A. Tucker and K. S. Thomas, 'Increasing Total Fiber Intake Reduces Risk of Weight and Fat Gains in Women', *J Nutr* 139, no. 3 (2009): 576–81.

60 A. Nilsson, E. Johansson, L. Ekström, and I. Björck, 'Effects of a Brown Beans Evening Meal on Metabolic Risk Markers and Appetite Regulating Hormones at a Subsequent Standardized Breakfast: A Randomized Cross-over Study', *PLoS ONE* 8, no. 4 (2013): e59985.

61 M. Zaraska, 'Bitter Truth', *New Scientist* 3032 (2015): 1–11.

62 H. Ilyasoğlu and N. A. Burnaz, 'Effect of Domestic Cooking Methods on Antioxidant Capacity of Fresh and Frozen Kale', *Int J Food Prop* 18 (2015): 1298–1305.

63 Y. Zhao, S. K. Du, H. Wang, and M. Cai, 'In Vitro Antioxidant Activity of Extracts from Common Legumes', *Food Chem* 152 (2014): 462–66.

64 H. C. Lin, N. A. Moller, M. M. Wolinsky, B. H. Kim, J. E. Doty, and J. H. Meyer, 'Sustained Slowing Effect of Lentils on Gastric Emptying of Solids in Humans and Dogs', *Gastroenterology* 102, no. 3 (1992): 787–92.

65 W. M. Fernando, J. E. Hill, G. A. Zello, R. T. Tyler, W. J. Dahl, and A. G. Van Kessel, 'Diets Supplemented with Chickpea or Its Main Oligosaccharide Component Raffinose Modify Faecal Microbial Composition in Healthy Adults', *Benef Microbes* 1, no. 2 (2010): 197–207.

66 M. Sajid and M. Ilyas, 'PTFE-Coated Non-stick Cookware and Toxicity Concerns: A Perspective', *Environ Sci Pollut Res Int* 24, no. 30 (2017): 23436–40.

67 Ibid.

68 D. T. Sugerman, 'Constipation', *JAMA* 310, no. 13 (2013): 1416.

69 D. P. Burkitt and P. Meisner, 'How to Manage Constipation with High-Fiber Diet', *Geriatrics* 34, no. 2 (1979): 33–35, 38–40.

70 A. M. Dias-Martins, K. L. F. Pessanha, S. Pacheco, J. A. S. Rodrigues, and C. W. P. Carvalho, 'Potential Use of Pearl Millet (*Pennisetum glaucum (L.) R. Br.*) in Brazil: Food Security, Processing, Health Benefits and Nutritional Products', *Food Res Int* 109 (2018): 175–86.

71 G. A. Annor, M. Marcone, E. Bertoft, and K. Seetharaman, 'In Vitro Starch Digestibility and Expected Glycemic Index of Kodo Millet (*Paspalum scrobiculatum*) as Affected by Starch–Protein–Lipid Interactions', *Cereal Chem* 90 (2013)0: 211–17.

72 J. Narayanan, V. Sanjeevi, U. Rohini, P. Trueman, and V. Viswanathan, 'Postprandial Glycaemic Response of Foxtail Millet Dosa in Comparison to a Rice Dosa in Patients with Type 2 Diabetes', *Indian J Med Res* 144, no. 5 (2016): 712–17.

73 H. Celik, N. Celik, A. Kocyigit, and M. Dikilitas, 'The Relationship between Plasma Aluminum Content, Lymphocyte DNA Damage, and Oxidative Status in Persons Using Aluminum Containers and Utensils Daily', *Clin Biochem* 45, no. 18 (2012): 1629–33.

74 D. Dordevic, H. Buchtova, S. Jancikova, et al., 'Aluminum Contamination of Food during Culinary Preparation: Case Study with Aluminum Foil and Consumers' Preferences', *Food Sci Nutr* 7, no. 10 (2019): 3349–60.

75 P. Pontieri, G. Mamone, S. De Caro, et al., 'Sorghum, a Healthy and Gluten-Free Food for Celiac Patients as Demonstrated by Genome, Biochemical, and Immunochemical Analyses', *J Agric Food Chem* 61, no. 10 (2013): 2565–71.

76 Joseph M. Awika, 'Sorghum: Its Unique Nutritional and Health-Promoting Attributes', in *Gluten-Free Ancient Grains: Cereals, Pseudocereals and Legumes*, ed. John R. N. Taylor and Joseph M. Awika (Cambridge, MA: Woodhead Publishing, 2017): 21–54.

77 S. Ragaee, E. S. M. Abdel-Aal, and M. Noaman, 'Antioxidant Activity and Nutrient Composition of Selected Cereals for Food Use', *Food Chem* 98, no. 1 (2006): 32–38.

78 L. De Morais Cardoso, S. S. Pinheiro, Martino, and H. M. Pinheiro-Sant'Ana, 'Sorghum (*Sorghum bicolor L.*): Nutrients, Bioactive Compounds, and Potential Impact on Human Health', *Crit Rev Food Sci Nutr* 57, no. 2 (2017): 372–90.

79 P. R. Shewry and S. Hey, 'Do "Ancient" Wheat Species Differ from Modern Bread Wheat in Their Contents of Bioactive Components?' *J Cereal Sci* 65 (2015): 236–43.

80 E. S. Abdel-Aal and I. Rabalski, 'Bioactive Compounds and Their Antioxidant Capacity in Selected Primitive and Modern Wheat Species', *Open Agr J* 2 (2008): 7–14.

81 D. Bazile, C. Pulvento, A. Verniau, et al., 'Worldwide Evaluations of Quinoa: Preliminary Results from Post International Year of Quinoa FAO Projects in Nine Countries', *Front Plant Sci* 7 (2016): 850.

82 A. M. Filho, M. R. Pirozi, J. T. Borges, H. M. Pinheiro Sant'Ana, J. B. Chaves, and J. S. Coimbra, 'Quinoa: Nutritional, Functional, and Antinutritional Aspects', *Crit Rev Food Sci Nutr* 57, no. 8 (2017): 1618–30.

83 D. Navarro-Perez, J. Radcliffe, A. Tierney, and M. Jois, 'Quinoa Seed Lowers Serum Triglycerides in Overweight and Obese Subjects: A Dose-Response Randomized Controlled Clinical Trial', *Curr Dev Nutr* 1, no. 9 (2017): e001321.

84 M. Romon, J. L. Edme, C. Boulenguez, J. L. Lescroart, and P. Frimat P, 'Circadian Variation of Diet-Induced Thermogenesis', *Am J Clin Nutr* 57, no. 4 (1993): 476–80.

85 M. L. Wahlqvist, 'Food Structure Is Critical for Optimal Health', *Food Funct* 7, no. 3 (2016): 1245–50.

86 F. S. Atkinson, K. Foster-Powell, and J. C. Brand-Miller, 'International Tables of Glycemic Index and Glycemic Load Values: 2008', *Diabetes Care* 31, no. 12 (2008): 2281–83.

87 A. R. Mackie, B. H. Bajka, N. M. Rigby, et al., 'Oatmeal Particle Size Alters Glycemic Index but Not as a Function of Gastric Emptying Rate', *Am J Physiol Gastrointest Liver Physiol* 313 no. 3 (2017): G239–46.

88 E. Petroff, E. F. Keane, E. D. Barr, et al., 'Identifying the Source of Perytons at the Parkes Radio Telescope', *Monthly Notices of the Royal Astronomical Society* 451, no. 4 (2015): 3933–40.

89 Z. O. Alhekail, 'Electromagnetic Radiation from Microwave Ovens', *J Radiol Prot* 21, no. 3 (2001): 251–58.

90 J. M. Hodgson, R. L. Prince, R. J. Woodman, et al., 'Apple Intake Is Inversely Associated with All-Cause and Disease-Specific Mortality in Elderly Women', *Br J Nutr* 115, no. 5 (2016;): 860–67.

91 N. P. Bondonno, C. P. Bondonno, L. C. Blekkenhorst, et al., 'Flavonoid-Rich Apple Improves Endothelial Function in Individuals at Risk for Cardiovascular Disease: A Randomized Controlled Clinical Trial', *Mol Nutr Food Res* 62, no. 3 (2018): 10.1002/mnfr.201700674.

92 M. Madero, J. C. Arriaga, D. Jalal, et al., 'The Effect of Two Energy-Restricted Diets, A Low-Fructose Diet versus a Moderate Natural Fructose Diet, on Weight Loss And Metabolic Syndrome Parameters: A Randomized Controlled Trial', *Metab Clin Exp* 60, no. 11 (2011): 1551–59.

93 H. Boeing, A. Bechthold, A. Bub, et al., 'Critical Review: Vegetables and Fruit in the Prevention of Chronic Diseases', *Eur J Nutr* 51, no. 6 (2012): 637–63.

94 A. Cassidy, 'Berry Anthocyanin Intake and Cardiovascular Health', *Mol Aspects Med* 61 (2018): 76–82.

95 H. Huang, G. Chen, D. Liao, Y. Zhu, and X. Xue, 'Effects of Berries Consumption on Cardiovascular Risk Factors: A Meta-analysis with Trial Sequential Analysis of Randomized Controlled Trials', *Sci Rep* 6 (2016): 23625.

96 Federal Institute for Risk Assessment, 'Cooking Spoons and Crockery MADE of Melamine Resin Are Not Suited for Microwaves and Cooking', Federal Ministry of Food, Agriculture and Consumer Protection, published December 5, 2011, available at https://www.bfr.bund.de/en/press_information/2011/11/cooking_spoons_and_crockery_made_of_melamine_resin_are_not_suited_for_microwaves_and_cooking-70465.html, accessed December 15, 2019.

97 Y. C. Tsai, C. F. Wu, C. C. Liu, et al., 'Urinary Melamine Levels and Progression of CKD', *Clin J Am Soc Nephrol* 14, no. 8 (2019): 1133–41.

98 C. D. Black, and P. J. O'Connor, 'Acute Effects of Dietary Ginger on Muscle Pain Induced by Eccentric Exercise', *Phytother Res* 24, no. 11 (2010) 1620–26.

99 P. B. Wilson, 'Ginger (*Zingiber officinale*) as an Analgesic and Ergogenic Aid in Sport: A Systemic Review', *J Strength Cond Res* 29, no. 10 (2015): 2980–95.

100 L. Biing-Hwan and J. Guthrie, 'Nutritional Quality of Food Prepared at Home and Away from Home, 1977–2008', US Department of Agriculture, Economic Research Service, Economic Information Bulletin 2012, 105 (Dec); M. Reicks, A. C. Trofholz, J. S. Stang, and M. N. Laska, 'Impact of Cooking and Home Food Preparation Interventions among Adults: Outcomes and Implications for Future Programs', *J Nutr Educ Behav* 46, no. 4 (2014): 259–76.

101 L. A. L. Soliah, J. M. Walter, and S. A. Jones, 'Benefits and Barriers to Healthful Eating: What Are the Consequences of Decreased Food Preparation Ability?' *American Journal of Lifestyle Medicine* 6, no. 2 (2012): 152–58.

102 R. Erlich, A. Yngve, and M. L. Wahlqvist, 'Cooking as a Healthy Behaviour', *Public Health Nutr* 15, no. 7 (2012) 1139–40.

103 K. Ried, 'Garlic Lowers Blood Pressure in Hypertensive Individuals, Regulates Serum Cholesterol, and Stimulates Immunity: An Updated Meta-analysis and Review', *J Nutr* 146, no. 2 (2016): 389S–96S.

104 E. Lissiman, A. L. Bhasale, and M. Cohen, 'Garlic for the Common Cold', *Cochrane Database Syst Rev* 4, no. 11 (2014): CD006206.

105 A. de Giorgio and J. Stebbing, 'Garlic: A Stake through the Heart of Cancer?' *Lancet Oncol* 17, no. 7 (2016): 879–80.

106 R. T. Kodali and G. D. Eslick, 'Meta-analysis: Does Garlic Intake Reduce Risk of Gastric Cancer?' *Nutr Cancer* 67, no. 1 (2015): 1–11.

107 F. Guarneri, C. Costa, S. P. Cannavò, et al., 'Release of Nickel and Chromium in Common Foods during Cooking in 18/10 (Grade 316) Stainless Steel Pots', *Contact Derm* 76, no. 1 (2017): 40–68.

108 C. Alves, A. Saleh, and H. Alaofè, 'Iron-Containing Cookware for the Reduction of Iron Deficiency Anemia among Children and Females of Reproductive Age in Low- and Middle-Income Countries: A Systematic Review', *PLoS ONE* 14, no. 9 (2019): e0221094.

109 S. A. Kulkarni, V. H. Ekbote, A. Sonawane, A. Jeyakumar, S. A. Chiplonkar, and A. V. Khadilkar, 'Beneficial Effect of Iron Pot Cooking on Iron Status', *Indian J Pediatr* 80, no. 12 (2013): 985–89.

110 B. J. Xu and S. K. Chang, 'Total Phenolic Content and Antioxidant Properties of Eclipse Black Beans (*Phaseolus vulgaris L.*) as Affected by Processing Methods', *J Food Sci* 73, no. 2 (2008): H19–27.

111 F. Natella, F. Belelli, A. Ramberti, and C. Scaccini, 'Microwave and Traditional Cooking Methods: Effect of Cooking on Antioxidant Capacity and Phenolic Compounds Content of Seven Vegetables', *J Food Biochem* 34 (2010): 796–810.

INDEX

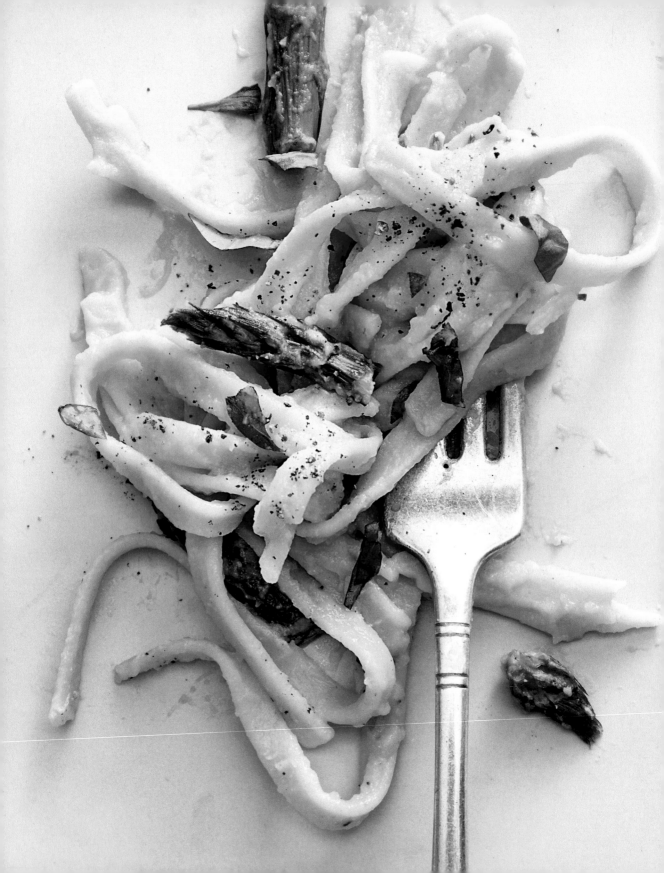